Planning Ahead
for Pregnancy

Planning Ahead for Pregnancy

DR. CHERRY'S GUIDE TO
HEALTH, FITNESS, AND FERTILITY

Sheldon H. Cherry, M.D.

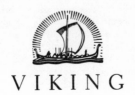

VIKING

VIKING
Viking Penguin Inc., 40 West 23rd Street,
New York, New York 10010, U.S.A.
Penguin Books Ltd, Harmondsworth,
Middlesex, England
Penguin Books Australia Ltd, Ringwood,
Victoria, Australia
Penguin Books Canada Limited, 2801 John Street,
Markham, Ontario, Canada L3R 1B4
Penguin Books (N.Z.) Ltd, 182–190 Wairau Road,
Auckland 10, New Zealand

First published in 1987 by Viking Penguin Inc.
Published simultaneously in Canada

Line illustrations on pages 95, 97, 197, 206 (top), and 207 are from the *Syntex Guide
to OB/GYN Conditions and Procedures* and are reproduced by
permission of Syntex Laboratories, Inc.

LIBRARY OF CONGRESS CATALOGING IN PUBLICATION DATA
Cherry, Sheldon H.
Planning ahead for pregnancy.
Includes index.
1. Prenatal care.   2. Pregnancy.   3. Women—Health
and hygiene.   4. Pregnant women—Health and hygiene.
5. Infertility, Human.   I. Title.
RG525.C6147 1987   618.2'4   86-40306
ISBN 0-670-80890-3

Printed in the United States of America by
R. R. Donnelley & Sons Company, Harrisonburg, Virginia
Set in Electra
Design by Mary A. Wirth

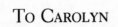

To Carolyn

Acknowledgments

I wish to thank the following people who aided in the preparation of this book:

Ellen Levine; Frank Bozzo for illustrations; Amanda Vaill; Alicia Fortenberry; Cara Cherry; Lisa Kaufman; Andre Smith

Valuable editorial assistance was given by Jennifer Kintzing Cadoff. To the Syntex Corporation, my thanks for allowing me to use their illustrations.

Contents

Introduction

We are in the middle of a revolution—a reproductive revolution. Basic "rules"—of family size, of when or whether to have children, of how couples organize their lives at home and at work—are being challenged. And we are faced with reverse challenges. Something seemingly as natural as being able to have a baby can no longer be taken for granted. The concept that the body will perform on demand is no longer valid in our complicated society. Planning ahead for childbirth has become important.

Women today are starting to recognize this. One young single woman said to me, "I don't have a boyfriend, much less a husband. Will I be able to conceive five—even ten—years from now if I do get married then?" Older women, facing a first pregnancy, ask me worriedly if a long-ago abortion or infection could have made them infertile. The concern, sometimes even fear, is there. And that's why I wrote this book, to tell every woman what I tell my patients: Just as working women spend time studying and preparing for careers, they can study and prepare for children. And in the same way an athlete strengthens her body to run a grueling marathon—with a plan of gradual physical training—a woman can ready her body so pregnancy will be as comfortable and healthy as possible.

There is no question that women are having children later in life. There has been a 15 percent rise in the birthrate among the thirty- to forty-five-year-olds, women who once were thought to be slightly beyond their childbearing years. One reason for this phenomenon is that 37 million postwar babies are now grown women—twenty-five to thirty-five years old. Their sheer numbers add clout to any changes in the way they, as a group, decide to lead their lives. As a broad generalization, these women marry later and hold off on having children until their educations are completed and their careers established. In addition, many single professional women and mothers of grown children are considering first or new pregnancies.

Another recent related trend is the move toward smaller families. The average number of children per family has dipped *below* two in the past ten years. Here, too, the reasons are complex. Obviously, the delay in the age of first pregnancies is a factor. If you have your first child at thirty-six, there is simply not as much time to have several more. A greater awareness of and concern about population problems may be another factor. Also, couples today have high expectations for their lives and the lives of their children; in a smaller family economic resources go further. And, of course, improved choices in contraception make it easier to plan for and limit the number of children a woman has.

In this time of fewer and later children, it has become even more important that both men and women take care of themselves from an early age. Without a doubt, active participation in your health and well-being is important to maintain fertility later in life. In our complex society, factors affecting future childbearing include environmental hazards such as x-rays; chemical pollutants in air, water, and food; smoking; exposure to both prescription and nonprescription drugs before (sometimes *years* before) and during pregnancy; and exposure to various illnesses such as rubella and toxoplasmosis that can harm a developing fetus. Informed prospective parents can avoid many potential threats and can do much to minimize the impact of dangers that prove to be unavoidable.

And that is exactly what this book is about: giving each couple who reads it the best possible chance of having a healthy baby when they decide to do so. This book will discuss how such diverse, important areas as family history, genetic problems, medical history, lifestyle, work environment, medications, eating habits, and even choice of contraceptive all have an impact on fertility.

It will be a reference book as well for couples with problems that may affect pregnancy. Medical counseling before pregnancy, of which this book plays just one part, can provide a realistic look at health status and at the general risks involved in a prospective pregnancy. Couples with high-risk conditions such as anemia, diabetes, or high blood pressure can thus make an informed decision. Now that we are able to diagnose over 200 genetic illnesses prior to delivery, it is important for couples to know whether they should consider genetic counseling prior to conception as well.

In addition, many couples (10 to 15 out of every 100) will have trouble conceiving. The incidence of infertility has increased in recent years because, as women have delayed their childbearing, their chances of having gynecologic problems have increased. This book will define and discuss the causes, diagnoses, and treatments of the most common fertility problems.

I will also take you from conception through the early phases of pregnancy, explaining how and when pregnancy is first detected, how the fetus grows and the mother's body changes, the tests your doctor may suggest, what can go wrong and what can be done about it.

In sum, this is a guide to planning ahead for a healthy child, no matter what stage of life you are in right now. It will help you protect your fertility until the time is right for childbearing, to prepare your body and mind once you're ready for pregnancy, to become pregnant, and to get your baby off to a healthy headstart.

Twenty years ago not many women thought of having a baby at thirty-five, even forty-five. But twenty years ago it didn't enter many women's heads to run twenty-six marathon miles, either. With the right knowledge, the right game plan, the right care and training of the body, both marathons and healthy pregnancies have become a reality for more women today than ever before.

PREPARING FOR A HEALTHY PREGNANCY: PRE- AND POSTCONCEPTION COUNSELING

As women, their goals, and their families have been changing, so medicine has been changing to keep pace. The goal of modern obstetrical care is to improve the quality of conception, pregnancy, and delivery so every baby will be born with the best possible chances for healthy physical and emotional development.

As long as ten years ago obstetricians began to think in terms of prevention of potential problems during and after delivery, by focusing on the identification and evaluation of high-risk pregnancies. They started to stress the need for evaluating a woman's health and heading off potential problems when, or even before, a new life was conceived.

Keeping in close touch with women just starting to plan for their pregnancies permits screening and timing of pregnancies in relation to the mother's overall and reproductive health.

The concept of high-risk pregnancy and special fetal care has produced a dramatic change, not only for women, but for their babies, too. The fetus has become the second patient, along with the mother, during pregnancy. Perinatology (the study and treatment of the fetus) and neonatology (the care of newborns) have developed as subspecialties within obstetrics and pediatrics. Modern perinatology probably dates from the early 1960s, when the first accurate intrauterine diagnostic test of fetal health was developed by Dr. William Liley in New Zealand.

By using amniocentesis (which involves drawing out, through a long needle inserted through the abdomen, a small amount of the amniotic fluid that surrounds the fetus) and analyzing various pigments in the fluid, Dr. Liley could determine the health status of a fetus with a blood disorder called "Rh incompatibility." Then he went one bold step further: He gave a transfusion of life-saving healthy blood to a sick fetus, while that unborn baby was still in the womb. The intrauterine fetal transfusion was a stunning first, and our fear of studying the intrauterine environment was dispelled. The field of perinatology took off in leaps and bounds.

These advances in the care of pregnant women, their fetuses, and their infants are, in all likelihood, responsible for the continued decreases in maternal and newborn death rates. Figure 1 shows infant mortality (death) rates for the years from 1930 to 1982. Figure 2 shows maternal mortality rates from 1950 to 1982.

But many problem areas remain in infant mortality. Deaths from congenital malformations (abnormalities with which a child is born), low birth weight, and poor growth while in the uterus have not really changed since 1979. Fortunately, these are areas where earlier and better care of mother and fetus can make a tremendous difference. Major problems could be avoided or minimized with greater availability of counseling prior to pregnancy and if the concept of prepregnancy planning and health care were more widespread.

You, the readers of this book, are the lucky ones. Your interest in knowing how to plan for pregnancy is a major factor in lowering your risks for certain problems over which you have some control. Even a little additional knowledge can lead you to ask the right questions, do the right things, in short, to have a better chance of having a healthy

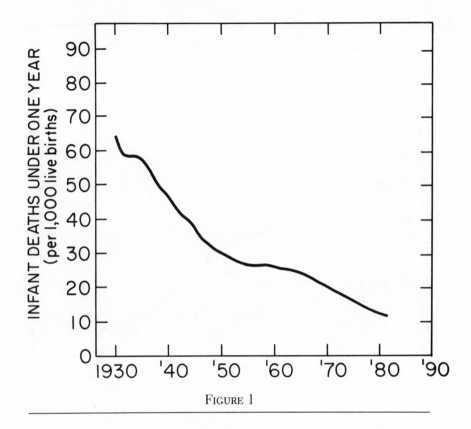

INFANT DEATHS UNDER ONE YEAR (per 1,000 live births)

1930 '40 '50 '60 '70 '80 '90

FIGURE 1

baby. The shift to later childbearing and the consequent high premium placed on each of these pregnancies are additional reasons for women to have the best quality of medical care possible before, during, and after pregnancy.

Women with diagnosed medical problems—diabetes, anemia, or high blood pressure, for example—have an even greater need for accurate medical advice prior to pregnancy. One of the purposes of this book is to provide some of that information. What exactly *are* the risks—to the woman, to her fetus? What can women do to reduce them? And what choices does a couple face for risks that can't be entirely predicted or controlled?

I have also tried to provide some reproductive counseling for couples who are at risk for genetic newborn problems or environment-related birth defects. Only your own doctor or genetic counselor can provide specific information about you and your partner as individuals. I can give general guidelines, discuss broad issues, and, I hope, convince every couple reading this book of the importance of getting the best and earliest medical advice possible.

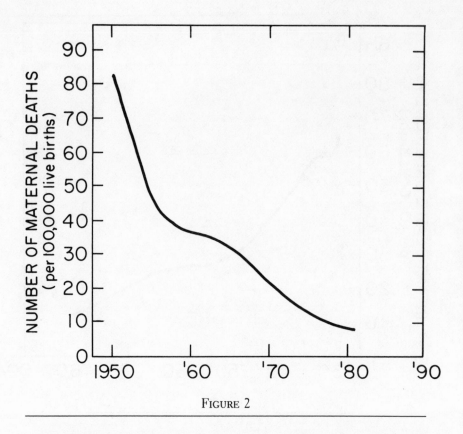

FIGURE 2

Many couples do already know the new responsibilities and possibilities of having a baby today. The term "reproductive anxiety" is a new one in our culture, denoting awareness of the important time prior to and during pregnancy. Knowledge can relieve unnecessary anxiety that isn't based on fact—since the facts stack up differently for each couple. It can also often relieve anxiety when there *is* a chance of a problem. Even difficult facts can be easier to accept and act on than living with gnawing, undefined fears. For example, 20 to 30 percent of pregnant women have some bleeding in early pregnancy. However, only 50 percent of these women will go on to have a miscarriage. Just knowing this can help reduce "reproductive anxiety."

Genetic counseling during pregnancy has become an integral part of most hospitals' departments of obstetrics and gynecology. Increased knowledge of human genetics as well as techniques such as amniocentesis and ultrasound have made it possible to diagnose many defects early in pregnancy and to predict the risk of recurrence in future pregnancies. (Chapter 14, "Genetic Counseling," discusses the conditions for which counseling is appropriate; Chapter 20, "Prenatal

Testing," covers amniocentesis and other tests done during pregnancy.)

Most medical centers already provide genetic counseling for women at risk for genetic disorders, and for women over thirty-five, or for families with known genetic problems. I recommend that this service be extended to include preconception counseling for women or couples with known *medical* problems that might affect conception, pregnancy, or birth. These would include: high blood pressure and heart disease; diabetes; certain maternal infections, such as herpes; exposure to certain drugs (both prescription and recreational); chronic pregnancy loss (several previous spontaneous miscarriages or abortions); DES exposure; history of small or low-birth-weight infants, or prematurity; risk of birth defects or mental retardation; long-term conditions such as epilepsy, chronic inflammatory bowel disease, neurological, blood, and lung disorders; serious underweight or overweight problems. (These topics will be discussed in detail in Chapter 21, "Medical Problems in Pregnancy.") All these conditions can benefit from preconception counseling and proper planning, and the baby will experience less fallout from the mother's health problems.

The bottom line, then, is that preparing for pregnancy really begins as soon as a teenager becomes a woman capable of bearing a child. From that time on her nutrition, exercise, choice of birth control, choice of sexual partners, and whether or not she smokes, drinks, or takes drugs may all have an impact on her future fertility. And once a woman actually decides to have children she can still make many health decisions that increase her odds of avoiding some problems altogether and minimizing others.

PART I

The Healthy Female

Introduction

Part I will review the female reproductive system, menstruation, and breast function and self-examination. I will also cover basic information on fitness and nutrition—what you need to know to prepare your body for pregnancy. These guidelines change once you become pregnant. (The specific aspects of diet and exercise relevant during gestation will be discussed in Part III.) Contraception information, also discussed with an eye toward a future pregnancy, completes this portion of the book.

So you may play an active role in your health care and develop a lifestyle that will guard your reproductive health, it is important that you understand both the anatomy of your reproductive system (what the various organs are, and where they are located) and its general physiology (how it works). And by understanding a bit of medical terminology—if only the "correct" name for body parts—you can also better understand what your physician says to you and, if you desire, shoulder some of the responsibility for health care decisions as well.

There are many myths and much misinformation about this area of the human body that are widely believed in our society. Knowing how to sift the facts from the half-truths is important. This kind of knowledge helps produce a healthy awareness of and joy in your body, for it is truly your most awesome possession. A knowledge of your body will also make you less anxious about things that are normal but disconcerting at first—like the odd lumpiness of your breasts when you learn to examine them—and less upset about things that go wrong, as they inevitably do—a skipped period, painful sex, a vaginal infection.

It is your body. Familiarity with its anatomy and how it works inspires confidence leading to a relaxed naturalness; this brings easy acceptance of and openness to your body's everyday functions, and to your sexual relationships as well.

1

The Female Reproductive System

Because women cannot easily see their external organs of reproduction, they may find it enlightening and useful to use a mirror to learn about themselves. "I felt kind of silly, sitting on the side of the tub with a mirror between my legs," one woman told me, "but after you gave me a mirror to look at my cervix during one of my checkups, that part of my body suddenly seemed real. So I wanted to become more familiar with other parts of me I can't usually see."

What the mirror will reveal, as shown in Figure 3, includes the minor and major labia (or lips of the vagina), the clitoris (an exquisitely sensitive organ protected by the mons veneris, the hairy pubic area, and the labia), the urethra (the tube urine travels through from the bladder), the opening of the vagina itself, the perineum (the area between the vagina and the anus), and the Bartholin glands.

The most prominent portions of the external genitalia are the labia. The labia majora, or large lips, are folded areas of skin covered with coarse, crinkly pubic hair and dotted with sweat glands. The labia minora, or small lips, lie within the labia majora, next to the opening of the vagina. The labia minora are covered by hairless skin with a large supply of sweat glands and nerves.

At the top of the external genitalia is the clitoris, sometimes covered by the folds of the labia. This organ has a very large blood supply and is made up of erectile tissue that has the ability to swell when blood rushes into it during sexual excitement—much like the male penis. The clitoris may be as long as an inch or as small as a quarter of an inch; but, again like a penis, size is not linked to the organ's ability to provide pleasure. The clitoris, large or small, is one of the most

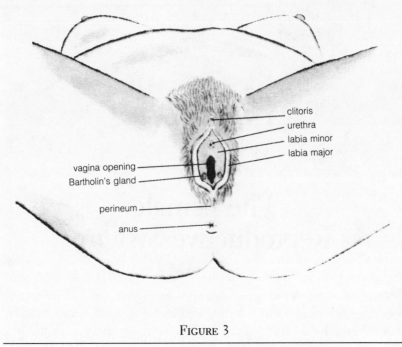

clitoris
urethra
labia minor
labia major

vagina opening
Bartholin's gland

perineum

anus

FIGURE 3

External organs of the female reproductive system

sensitive areas of a woman's body because of its abundant network of nerves.

The urethra, through which urine exits the body, is a very small opening between the vaginal opening and the clitoris. Because of its proximity to the vagina and the clitoris the delicate tissue of the urethra occasionally becomes irritated during vigorous sex. Urination may be slightly painful just after intercourse, as the urine passes by the over-rubbed area. (This is different from and more temporary than the pain of a urinary tract infection, which is discussed in Chapter 7, "Common Infections.")

The hymen, a thin fold of membrane at the mouth of the vagina, usually has a small opening that stretches to accommodate a penis without too much difficulty the first time a woman has sex. But more extreme situations are not uncommon. The opening may be small enough to require a fair amount of tearing or stretching in order to allow sexual intercourse. Or it may be large enough to be no obstacle at all, even in a virgin.

The Bartholin glands, two groups of glandular tissue along either side of the vaginal opening, produce mucus that contributes to vaginal lubrication during sex. Generally, the glands themselves are not visible;

only the fluid they produce reveals their presence. However, occasionally one of them becomes infected and can swell to a quite prominent and painful lump.

The vagina, or birth canal, extends inward from the external genitals to connect to the inner reproductive organs. When you are standing, the three- to six-inch-long vagina is at about a 45-degree angle to the horizontal, slanting up toward the small of your back. This flat, skin-lined tube has an extraordinary capacity to expand during both sexual intercourse and childbirth. After sex, it will return to its earlier size, although the stretching of childbearing tends to leave the vagina permanently enlarged. Usually this enlargement or change will not interfere with sexual pleasure for either partner. The vagina is not nearly as sensitive as the clitoris, although deep pressure is readily felt. There is an area on the upper wall of the vagina, about one inch in from the opening, popularly dubbed the "G spot" or Grafenberg spot. According to some experts, this area has a greater concentration of nerves and, thus, has a greater importance in sexual excitement and orgasm. Women who have increased sensitivity in this area can generally point to the spot quite easily.

The internal pelvic organs (Figures 4 and 5)—uterus, or womb, vagina, rectum, and bladder—are all supported in the pelvis by muscles and ligaments. There is a series of interlocking muscles that are attached to the side walls of the pelvis, and meet in the middle to support the organs. These muscles can sometimes be injured during childbearing, which can lead to certain physical problems years later. Modern obstetrical management of birth and delivery has evolved to minimize the chance of damage to these important muscles.

The uterus is divided into two areas. The neck of the uterus, where it opens into the vagina, is called the cervix. By inserting a finger into the vagina, the cervix can be felt as a thumb-tip-sized bump protruding into the top of the vagina. The fist-sized body of the uterus, the fundus, is supported by pelvic muscles as well as ligaments extending from the sides of the uterus to the pelvic bones. In the cervix there is a small channel called the "cervical canal," through which sperm travel in search of an egg to fertilize and out of which menstrual fluid flows. During the delivery of a child the cervix expands, or dilates, to about nine or ten centimeters (about three to four inches), allowing the infant to pass from the uterus into the vagina, and, finally, to be born.

Occasionally women are born with an unusually shaped uterus. The most common is the so-called bicornuate or double uterus, with a wall

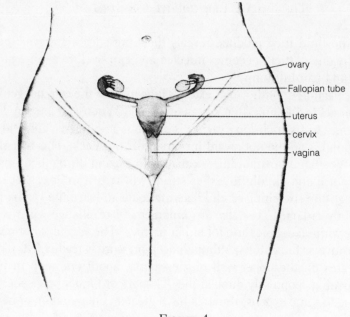

FIGURE 4

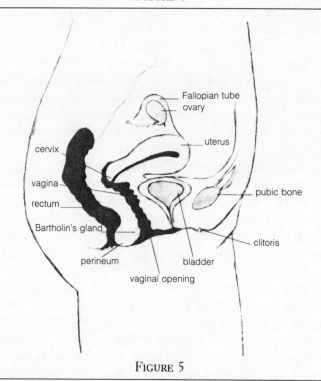

FIGURE 5

Internal organs of the female reproductive system

of tissue dividing it down the center. Most uterine abnormalities, including this one, are relatively minor, and do not affect menstruation, conception, or pregnancy. (Situations that may cause problems will be discussed in greater detail in Chapters 19 and 22, "Problems of Early Pregnancy" and "The Causes of Infertility.")

The inside lining of the uterus is called the "endometrium." Fluctuations in various hormone levels in the bloodstream during the menstrual cycle cause this tissue to change in a predictable way. And it is the endometrial tissue that, if a woman doesn't conceive, sloughs off, resulting in what you know as the menstrual flow. If, on the other hand, a fertilized egg implants in the uterus, the endometrium is the source of nutrients and blood for the developing pregnancy.

On either side of the uterus is one Fallopian tube, each about four to five inches long—the path an egg must travel from ovary to uterus. It is actually in the Fallopian tubes that egg and sperm meet and life begins. The Fallopian tubes are not just passive pipes for this process. They are, for example, active participants in retrieving an egg as it pops from the ovary, by means of thousands of softly waving flaglike "fimbria" that sprout from the tubes' ends. The tubes are lined with millions of tiny hairs called "cilia," which then sweep the egg along its path into the waiting endometrial lining of the uterus. The walls of the tubes are also capable of muscular contractions, whose function is not clear. These contractions may aid sperm or egg migration. (Changes in tubal function can lead to "ectopic," or "tubal," pregnancy, discussed in Chapters 7 and 19, "Common Infections" and "Problems of Early Pregnancy.")

The two ovaries—a woman's basic sex organs—lie one on each side of the uterus and are held in place by fibrous ligaments. The ovaries produce the essential female hormones, estrogen and progesterone, as well as the eggs from which pregnancy can occur. Each amazingly efficient ovary is about the size of a large plum: When even as much as 95 percent of ovarian tissue is removed, normal menstruation and pregnancy can, and do, still take place. Every woman is born with all the eggs she will ever have (about a million) already in her ovaries; by contrast, a man's testicles constantly manufacture new sperm. Female eggs simply lie in waiting in the essentially dormant ovaries until puberty. By the time the ovaries come to life and the menstrual cycle begins, probably 500,000 viable eggs remain. During a woman's reproductive years only a tiny proportion of these eggs ever have a chance at being released during ovulation. About 50 eggs start ripening each month, but usually only one of these is released at ovulation. The rest simply waste away. Although having so many extra eggs may seem inefficient, it is this multiple backup system that allows this cycle to be so steady and dependable over thirty-plus years.

The Menstrual Cycle

While the ovary is the central organ of the reproductive system, it is the menstrual cycle that is this system's reason for being. Each month this intricate, delicately balanced process is set in motion again. Each month the body readies itself for pregnancy.

At menarche, which is the onset of a woman's fertile years, ovulation occurs for the first time. Today this happens most often between the ages of ten and sixteen. In comparison with other mammals, menstrual function comes relatively late in humans, delaying the age at which we can reproduce and increasing the relative time we spend as children. Over the last 100 years, menarche has tended to come earlier and earlier in humans—the average age has declined by about four months every ten years. The trend to earlier puberty is probably linked to the worldwide movement toward better standards of hygiene and diet. This may not be the whole story, but evidence supporting this theory exists today: Women from areas of high socioeconomic development menstruate sooner than women in world poverty areas. Good nutrition seems to influence the development of the part of the brain called the "hypothalamus," and the hypothalamus is the trigger area that sets off ovulation and menstruation.

Heredity is another major influence in the timing of puberty and menarche. The age at which your mother, grandmother, or sister started menstruating is likely to be echoed in your body. In fact, other reproductive cycle patterns, including the menopause age, are often paralleled in the women in a family as well.

Whatever age menstruation starts, the first year or so tends to be quite irregular, as the body concentrates on getting the kinks out of the system. The process of a normal ovulatory cycle involves a complex interrelationship between the pituitary gland of the brain, the uterus, and the ovaries. Although this varies from individual to individual, by the age of eighteen most women are ovulating regularly and have developed the ability to become pregnant.

The menstrual cycle itself can be broken down into three distinct phases:

1. The preovulation phase, characterized by secretion of estrogen by the ovaries to trigger a buildup of the lining of the uterus;
2. The postovulation phase, which involves the secretion of progesterone from the ovary to make the lining of the uterus ready for a fertilized egg to implant; and
3. The menstrual phase, which, if there is no pregnancy, is the dismantling and discarding of the endometrium.

Menstruation results when the body fails to achieve pregnancy. The lining of the uterus, so meticulously prepared to be the best possible environment for a fertilized egg, must simply be sloughed off and expelled from the body. But the reproductive system immediately starts to prepare for the next ovum: The reconstruction of the endometrium begins immediately after menstruation ends. And so it goes, month after month, throughout the reproductive life of a woman. Except, of course, during pregnancy, and sometimes during breastfeeding as well.

About three-quarters of the lining of the uterine surface is shed during menstruation. Regeneration occurs from the remaining bottommost one-quarter. The amount of blood lost during menstruation varies from woman to woman and also from cycle to cycle, ranging on average from one to six ounces, a small amount that most women will not miss at all, since the body quickly produces new red blood cells to compensate. Think of it this way: Blood donors give about a pint—which is sixteen ounces—of blood with no ill effects. Nonetheless, it is important to get adequate iron in the diet so that, over time, the body's stores are not depleted. This is especially true for women who bleed heavily. They, in fact, might want to ask their gynecologist to do a simple blood test to check for anemia whenever they are in the office for a routine checkup.

As soon as menstruation is complete the pituitary gland in the brain alerts an ovary to start ripening a new egg, by releasing a hormone called "follicle stimulating hormone" or FSH. (The cells surrounding a developing egg are called the "follicle.") The follicle is also in charge of producing the primary female hormone, estrogen, which promotes the regrowth of the uterine lining. During the first two weeks of the cycle, the amount of estrogen churned out by the follicle gradually increases. When it builds to a critical level, it gives a feedback signal to the pituitary gland in the brain, which then knows it's time to release another hormone, called "luteinizing hormone" (or LH). It is LH's task to stimulate the egg's release from the now mature follicle—the event known as ovulation.

Ovulation and the few days which follow it are the period of highest fertility. Many factors affect the time of ovulation, some of them not, as yet, completely understood. But, at base, the production of an adequate amount of estrogen, followed by the production of LH, is definitely required. In some mammals ovulation can be triggered after intercourse or, simply, sexual excitement. Ovulation can follow every sexual act in the rabbit, which accounts for its legendary high fertility rate. In the human female, however, ovulation is cyclic and is not stimulated by external influences. In fact, human ovulation seems to work in the other direction: Instead of being triggered, it can be *inhibited* by external forces—stress, weight loss, or strenuous exercise.

Following ovulation the egg is picked up by tiny waving flags of tissue (fimbria) at the end of the Fallopian tubes and swept along toward the endometrium. The area from which the egg was released in the ovary changes character: It is no longer an estrogen-producing follicle; it now becomes the "corpus luteum," and produces progesterone, the second hormone of the menstrual cycle. The role of this hormone is to encourage the estrogen-thickened endometrium to develop a lush, so-called secretory lining, rich in sugar and enzymes that can nourish a fertilized egg. The blood supply to the uterine lining also increases, so that the endometrial tissues can become a healthy environment for the awaited fertilized egg. If, after all this preparation, fertilization does not take place, the production of progesterone by the corpus luteum wanes, and the corpus luteum itself begins to disappear. And, with no progesterone to support it, the lining of the endometrium starts to shed and menstruation begins. The unused egg simply dries up and is expelled, invisibly, with the menstrual flow.

But even as all that happens, the body is poised to start all over again. The end of the cycle is not just an ending, it's a new beginning as well. That fact is reflected in our terming: "Day 1" of the menstrual cycle is the first day of bleeding which has resulted from the previous cycle.

MENSTRUAL VARIATION

The time from day 1 of one cycle to day 1 of the next is usually about 28 days. Perfectly normal cycles, however, can range between 23 and 35 days. Cycles shorter than 21 days or longer than 38 should be evaluated by your doctor. There is most often nothing wrong; but when something does occur out of normal range, it's a good idea for your doctor to keep an eye on it. Some women ovulate only every other month, for example, and may, then, have a 60-day cycle. If that's what is "normal" for them, there's really nothing wrong with a two-month cycle. The only problem is that it may be more difficult for such women to become pregnant, since they ovulate only about half as often as other women.

In fact, so many things can upset the cycle that it sometimes seems surprising that we can determine what a "normal" one is at all. Irregular periods are common, as we have said, for a year or so after menarche. The same is true in the years before menopause, the average age of which is fifty-one. Weight gain or weight loss, excessive emotional or physical stress, various types of illnesses, even changes in time zone can upset menstrual rhythms even during the typically steadier middle reproductive years.

Regular, vigorous exercise is another common culprit in irregular cycles. Occasionally, menstrual periods stop completely—a condition known as "amenorrhea" (which means the absence of menstruation). Exactly how exercise has its impact on the cycle is not fully understood. However, several factors are being studied, including the loss of body fat, stress, and changes in the amount of body hormones. Irregularities in menstrual cycles occur from running more often than from any other sport. Women who exceed twenty to thirty miles per week seem to be particularly at risk. From what is known at this point, however, exercise-induced menstrual changes appear to be completely reversible: When the mileage in running is reduced, for example, normal cycles simply resume as if nothing had interrupted them.

Another thing some women are concerned about is the number of days their menstrual flow lasts. Here, again, there is a wide range of normal. The average woman will bleed for about three to five days. However, some will bleed for as many as six or as few as two. Sometimes women will have spotting for a day or two prior to the onset of flow. This, too, is considered normal. In addition, some women have a small amount of midcycle bleeding, sometimes accompanied by a bit of twinge-y cramping, approximately two weeks before their periods. This bleeding is associated with ovulation and is nothing to be concerned about. It usually lasts only one day and involves a very small amount of blood.

Occasionally women don't start to menstruate during their teenage years. This condition is called "primary amenorrhea," to signify that periods never began, in contrast to "secondary amenorrhea," which is when cycles stop after there have been some regular periods. A woman not menstruating by age sixteen or seventeen should see her doctor. Women who are just starting to have periods find there is much variation in duration and frequency, though this will eventually settle down into a somewhat regular pattern. Once that happens, a woman who misses periods frequently or who has stopped menstruating for more than three months should see her doctor too. (Sooner if there's any chance of the number-one reason for amenorrhea—pregnancy!) As women approach menopause, the pattern may change again. Periods tend to become less regular and less frequent as the ovaries reach the end of their working years. These changes are not anything to worry about as long as there are no other symptoms, such as excessive menstrual flow or bleeding between periods.

There is a general misconception that women who start to menstruate earlier will probably stop menstruating at a younger age. In fact, the opposite is more likely: There is a general tendency for women with early menarche to have later menopause. However, probably the best clue as to when menopause will occur is the age at which it occurred in other women in your family, since most women tend to have the same menstrual patterns as their mothers and grandmothers.

A Note on Toxic Shock Syndrome

The choice of vaginal tampons versus sanitary napkins is a personal one. However, the recent Toxic Shock Syndrome scare has alerted us to the need for changing tampons frequently. Toxic shock is a rare problem, characterized by a fever, rash, and diarrhea. Some physicians advise the use of tampons only during the day and the use of sanitary pads at night. Any fever during menstruation should be reported to your physician. Another rare cause of toxic shock is the contraceptive sponge. The sponge should not be left in place longer than 24 hours, and should not be used at all during menstruation.

The Vaginal Discharge

Soon after the onset of their first period, most women will also notice a different type of vaginal discharge. This creamy effusion helps to keep the vagina moist, pliable, and self-cleaning, and acts as a natural protection against some kinds of bacteria. Special glands in the cervix are prompted by the release of the hormone estrogen to produce mucus, which is perceived as a vaginal discharge. The amount of this discharge varies greatly from woman to woman, and for any one woman during her menstrual cycle. The maximum amount of flow is apparent around midcycle (when some women find it profuse enough to warrant the use of a mini-pad); the minimum just before menstruation. In addition, the character of the mucus changes during the month. At peak fertility, midcycle, it is silky and elastic, and actually assists sperm in their quest for an egg by making passage through the cervical canal easier. At less fertile times it becomes thicker, pastier, more difficult for sperm to penetrate.

Vaginal discharge can be affected by emotional and medical conditions. Drugs such as the birth control pills change the amount and character of cervical mucus, and sexual excitement, of course, results in an effusion of its own. Most of the slippery wetness brought on by arousal is from vaginal "sweating"—fluid literally is exuded through the walls of the vagina, much as your skin exudes sweat in hot weather. In addition, the cells that line the vagina are constantly shedding and being replaced by new ones, just like the skin. This keeps the vagina healthy and clean, and contributes somewhat to the everyday, non-arousal discharge.

Although it sounds odd, in a healthy vagina there are actually many types of bacteria. Again, a parallel can be drawn with the skin: On healthy skin various types of bacteria live in harmony with your body. These bacteria, in the vagina or on skin, don't cause infections under normal conditions. In fact, their presence actually helps create an environment in which "outside invader" bacteria cannot gain a foothold.

Normal vaginal discharge should be clear or slightly cloudy, due to its makeup of vaginal cells, bacteria, and mucus secretions from the cervix. It has a distinct although not disagreeable odor. Occasionally, a normal discharge may be yellow. A marked change in vaginal discharge may indicate a problem: A disagreeable odor, a heavy discharge with an unusual color, a discharge that is irritating or itchy to the external organs, should all be an alert to see your doctor. (Vaginal infections will be discussed in greater detail in Chapter 7, "Common Infections.")

DOUCHING AND FEMININE SPRAYS

The process of douching (gently flushing the vagina with various liquid concoctions, which are held in a bag, via a tube inserted into the vagina) has been used for many centuries and for many reasons, some of which make little sense in terms of our current understanding of the reproductive system. Today, douching is used in an attempt by women to eliminate disagreeable odors and occasionally by physicians to treat local infections in the vagina. Basically, however, a woman does not need to douche as a regular part of her personal hygiene. As I have explained, the normal secretions in the vagina are specifically designed to keep it healthy and free of infection, and they do so very efficiently. Any infection the vagina can't handle alone is not likely to be helped by a nonprescription douche liquid anyway. The vagina, in short, does not normally require any assistance in doing its job. Periodic douching once or twice a week will not usually be harmful and may be psychologically comforting to some women. Excessive douching, on the other hand, can actually interfere with the body's ability to keep the vagina healthy, and make infection more, not less, likely. Excessive douching can lead to problems in conceiving by washing out the important cervical mucus at ovulation time. (Douching, by the way, is absolutely *not* an effective means of birth control.)

The concept of odor of the vagina is very subjective; problems can, perhaps, be more imagined than real. In most healthy women the odors in the vaginal area are probably due more to sweating and from wearing tight-fitting clothes like jeans and pantyhose than from secretions. In these cases douching is unnecessary, since the source of the odor is not in the vagina. Simple washing of the external genital area with soap and warm water is usually all that is required as treatment.

All the douches that line the shelves, with their varying amounts of perfumes, have one thing in common: They are all acidic, like the healthy vagina. The simple, old-fashioned, standby vinegar douche (consisting of two tablespoons of white vinegar to one quart of warm water) produces an acid solution similar to that of the normal vagina. If you do want to douche occasionally, it is best to ask your physician to recommend a specific acidity and type of douche.

Feminine hygiene sprays are another frequently promoted product aimed at women. Many of these advertisements pander to women's insecurities about disease, lack of cleanliness, and odor. According to the ads, these sprays will make you smell like a rose garden (or a bowl of strawberries) instead of a woman. In reality, the artificial perfumes and preservatives in the sprays may produce allergic reactions and tissue irritation. If you are healthy, a daily bath or shower is all that is necessary to keep this area clean. If you have an offensive or unusual odor due to an infection, you need a physician to diagnose the ailment and clear it up.

In our culture there are still many myths, taboos, and misunderstandings circulating regarding menstruation. In the past, thinking about menstruation was clouded with feelings of shame and fears of uncleanliness—the residue of scientific ignorance and religious and cultural taboos. Unfortunately, many young women are still instilled with a sense of shame and secrecy even before they get their first periods. A fifteen-year-old told me recently, "I was so excited about 'becoming a woman' I rushed to the living room to tell my father and my brothers. They could hardly look at me for embarrassment! I didn't know what I'd done wrong. I was so hurt! My dad won't let me roughhouse with my brothers now because I'm too grown up. It felt like punishment."

Myths and folklore proliferate where education is lacking. Many women to this day still believe that they cannot swim or take a bath while they are menstruating. Some still believe that if a woman misses a menstrual period, she may become "sick" because of a buildup of poisons or toxins in her blood. In other words, menstruation is believed to be necessary to get rid of dirty products that accumulate. However, there is no truth in this concept; a skipped period has no impact on your general health. The only reason a missed period is important is that it may signal either pregnancy or that something may be wrong with your physical health or emotional well-being.

Fortunately, many women now see menstruation as a unique female experience, feel joy and wonder at the astonishing complexity and delicate balance of the cycle, and understand its relationship to the miraculous process of reproduction. This often brings them an increase in respect for themselves. With better education, the embarrassment and guilt some women still associate with menstruation will slowly disappear.

2

The Breast

During pregnancy, and while a woman is breastfeeding, she is constantly reminded of the breasts' primary purpose: to provide an infant with nourishment, a means of survival. But at other times the breasts can also be a major source of anxiety, and not just because some women fear theirs don't meet the current requirements of fashion. Breast cancer is the leading cause of cancer deaths in women.

One of the reasons the fear of cancer looms so large is that women are constantly exhorted by their physicians to examine their breasts— because concerned doctors know firsthand what a life-saving difference this simple habit can make. But women are often intimidated by their unfamiliarity with their breasts. Odd, but true. For all the attention breasts get in our society, women may still not feel comfortable pressing, squeezing, and prodding them. The other major reason women may be loath to perform their monthly self-exam is illogical but persuasive: If they look for a lump, maybe they'll find one.

BASIC BREAST ANATOMY

Beneath the smooth skin of the breast lie lumpy masses of tissue called "lobules." These are the basic working units of the breast. Within each lobule is a gland called an "aveolus" and a duct leading from that gland to the nipple. The aveolus is the breast's milk-producing area. The duct is the conduit that transfers the milk to the nipple for release. The milk-producing system receives its main stimulation for growth and development around puberty, when the hormone estrogen is produced by the ovaries. Once fully developed, the breasts are ready for milk production, but produce no milk until the many physical and hormonal changes of pregnancy signal a need for lactation. Breasts come in all sizes and shapes, but the ability to breast-feed is not affected by these variations. Breastfeeding can be successfully accomplished by most women.

Breasts are very sensitive to the hormones estrogen and progesterone, whose monthly ebb and flow accounts for the changes that occur during the menstrual cycle and during pregnancy. Your breasts may swell premenstrually from rising progesterone and estrogen levels. During pregnancy breasts will enlarge and prepare to produce milk.

SELF-EXAMINATION OF THE BREAST

Although a woman's physician will carefully examine her breasts each time she comes in for a checkup, it is critically important that she get in the habit of examining her own breasts once each month. The best time is the week after your period—the breasts are least likely to be swollen, lumpy, or sore at this time. As you do this, you will gradually become comfortable with the normal anatomy and shape of your breasts, so that you can feel any changes that may occur. Once you get to this point, your doctor is no longer the number-one authority on your breasts and what they feel like. You are.

The suspicious changes you're training your fingers to be on the lookout for include lumps, bumps, discharge, and irregularities. It is extremely important to keep in mind that even if you do find something unusual, odds are it is *not* malignant. However, any change in your breasts should be brought to your doctor's attention immediately.

Step one in your exam is to stand naked in front of a mirror, with your arms hanging loosely at your sides. Look for any puckering or dimpling of the skin of the breasts or retraction of the nipples, or changes in the breast size or shape. Now rest your hands on your hips and press your hands into your sides, and look for the same things. Repeat your scrutiny again, arms held high overhead.

Next, lie flat on your back, placing your left hand under your head, and, with the flat pads of the fingers of your other hand, gently but firmly press your left breast. Use small, circular motions of your fingertips to move the skin over the tissue that lies beneath it. These circular movements must be repeated over every inch of breast. One way to examine the entire breast is outlined in Figure 6. Different people feel comfortable using different patterns. Some doctors, and

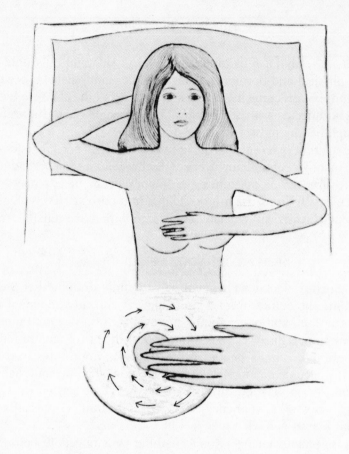

FIGURE 6

Technique for self-examination of the breasts. In the supine position with one hand elevated, the other hand examines the breast with small circular motions.

women, prefer to move over the breast in concentric circles—starting at the breast's outer perimeter and moving in toward the nipple about an inch at a time. Others divide the breast into imaginary quarters, or quadrants, and check each one by one. The pattern doesn't matter as long as the entire breast, including the tissue tucked away up almost into the armpit, is checked. Examine the nipple area in the same way, and gently squeeze the nipple to see if any fluid comes out. After examining the left breast, put your right arm up over your head, and repeat your exam on the right breast. You can also do a less thorough, but still helpful, exam in the shower or tub. Running your hands over the breasts is quite easy when the skin is slippery with water and soap.

Many women have lumpy breasts, especially in the week or so before menstruation. What you are looking for is something new or unusual. If you become familiar with the normal size, contour, and consistency of your own breasts it will help you a great deal. These factors vary tremendously with each woman. But they should not vary significantly with the same woman from one month to the next.

For all that a breast exam is worth to women's health, it can only reveal so much by itself. Finding a lump is only a signal for further tests. It's not a diagnosis—or anywhere close—all by itself. There are approximately four benign lesions found for every malignant one. Even doctors find it impossible to tell simply by feeling it whether a small mass is benign or malignant. There are clues—its shape, size, location, relative hardness, and whether or not it is moveable—that point in one direction or the other. But diagnosis will require more tests— maybe mammography, needle aspiration, or surgical biopsy. However, try not to panic. The chances of a single lump being malignant are far less than the chance that it is benign, especially in women under the age of fifty.

☐ *Benign breast diseases* may be noncancerous growths of many different kinds. Sometimes the worst thing about them is the diagnostic process and the anxiety that occurs before the diagnosis is certain.

Fibrocystic disease of the breast is the most common type of breast problem. It is also called "chronic mastitis," "cystic mastitis," and "cystic disease of the breast." By whatever name, this problem is, unfortunately, often difficult to treat. There are two major types of fibrocystic disease. One is the generally painful, swollen, nodular breast. The other, milder form involves one (or just a few) small, cystlike swelling. Fibrocystic disease occurs only during the menstrual years, often appearing in the early twenties and thirties and slowly disappearing after menopause. During pregnancy it also seems to improve.

The symptoms are pain and tenderness in the breast, sometimes severe enough to prevent sleep. Some women cannot even lie face down, especially during their menstrual periods, when the pain is usually worst. Diagnosis is usually made by the symptoms and their predictable recurrence with each menstrual cycle. Most of the time this condition does not require treatment, other than pain medication for relief. However, if pain is very severe and persistent, small doses of diuretics, progesterone, or vitamin B complex may be of help. While all-over tenderness and lumpiness of both breasts is common, the upper and outer quadrant of the breast (nearest the armpit) tends to be the hardest hit.

With the milder form of fibrocystic disease there is only a single cyst, or at most a few small cysts, in one area of the breast. This tends to swell before menstruation. These cysts usually cause no pain, but— while this is an undeniable plus—the flip side is that a painless cyst is very difficult to differentiate from cancer. Physical examination usually reveals a clearly defined, round, and moveable mass. The doctor may insert a small needle into the lump to try to "aspirate" it, or suck out the fluid. If fluid can be removed, this means the lump *was* benign and also cures the cyst. However, if fluid cannot be aspirated, the fluid that comes out is bloody, or there is a firm mass left after the fluid is drained, then further tests are in order. Mammography and sonography (ultrasound) can give clues to the diagnosis of these lumps; surgical excision (usually a very minor procedure) is often necessary when a firm decision can't be made otherwise.

Fibroadenomas are small, benign, encapsulated tumors that appear shortly after puberty. They can occur throughout the twenties, but become more rare as women age. These small masses may not disappear after menopause; occasionally they become calcified, or hardened into rocklike lumps. Fibroadenomas cause no symptoms and are usually discovered by accident or during a breast self-examination. These lumps are characteristically small, solid, firm, well-circumscribed, and mobile. Usually, larger fibroadenomas will be surgically removed. Smaller ones can simply be watched; they are very slow-growing. About half the time a woman will have more than one.

Another disorder is *inflammatory mastitis*. This is a bacterial infection in the milk ducts which requires treatment with antibiotics and soaks. Its symptoms—swelling, tenderness, and redness—can occur at any time, not just during pregnancy or nursing, and will subside with treatment.

The mainstays of detection and treatment of breast disease are self-examination, physical examination by your physician, and mammography. Mammography alone does not replace careful physical examination. In fact, routine use of mammography is not usually recommended before age forty. However, when a mass is discovered or a woman has breast cancer in her family, earlier mammography may be suggested. (The recommendations of the American Cancer Society are outlined on page 24.)

☐ *Cancer of the breast* is the most common malignancy in women in this country. Its peak occurrence is around menopause. Five percent of women will eventually be diagnosed as having cancer of the breast.

Certain factors have been related to breast cancer. The genetic influence is clear: A woman's chance of getting breast cancer is four times greater if her mother had it. Other fairly clear factors relating to breast cancer include a high-fat diet, the use of estrogens, and the failure to nurse or become pregnant.

The role of estrogen in development of breast cancer is suggested by the fact that women who have had their ovaries removed are less likely to get breast cancer. Women who get breast cancer tend to have a longer span of menstrual years, with an early onset of puberty and a late menopause. There is some evidence that breast cancer may be induced in some susceptible women by prolonged administration of estrogens.

Breast cancer does tend to appear with greater frequency in women who are unmarried, who have borne few or no children, and who did not nurse those who were born. If there is a history of previous cystic disease of the breast, cancer is four times more common. It is also more common in the areas of the breast where cystic disease is more common, namely the upper outer quadrant.

Trauma to the breast has nothing to do with causing cancer. However, by injuring yourself, you may accidentally discover an abnormality that was already in the breast.

Although symptoms of breast cancer are minimal, early diagnosis is the mainstay of successful treatment. Breast exams, then, must be the first step. Treatment itself depends on a number of factors such as the woman's age, health, the biological nature of the tumor, and the extent of the disease.

Since breast cancer is not preventable, it is critical to try to diagnose it early, when cure rates are very high. Some women are so overcome with fear at the discovery of a nodule that they keep its presence a secret from their families and their doctors. Sometimes they even deny its presence to themselves. This attitude unfortunately contributes to keeping the death rate from breast cancer high among American women.

Careful monthly self-examination is simple, inexpensive, and effective for early diagnosis and treatment of breast cancer, and has saved thousands of lives. Since early breast cancer has a cure rate in excess of 80 percent, self-examination may someday save your life. Until we find a cure for breast cancer it is our best hope for minimizing death and disability. The fear of discovering a lump is understandable; risking your life because of the fear is not. And, like most scary things in life, when faced head on the fear retreats a bit and a sense of accomplishment and control over your life takes its place.

MAMMOGRAPHY

Mammography—an x-ray of the breast that requires a very low dose of radiation—has established itself as the primary tool for the early medical detection of breast cancer. It is so sensitive that cancer can be diagnosed before the victim can feel its effects.

The American Cancer Society has issued the following recommendations:

- A "baseline" mammogram (the standard against which subsequent mammograms can be compared) for women ages thirty-five to thirty-nine
- Mammography every one to two years for women forty to forty-nine, depending on risk factors and findings
- Mammography every year for women ages fifty and over, whether or not they have any suspicious symptoms.

Discuss these recommendations with your physician.

3

Exercise and Diet
Before Pregnancy

"A sound mind in a sound body" (*mens sana in corpore sano*, Juvenal, *Satire X*) has been a medical ideal since ancient times. The phrase was originally intended simply to emphasize the importance of a balanced concern toward physical plus mental health. However, as scientists continue to unravel the layers of interdependence between these two delicately entwined parts of ourselves, it becomes clearer that a strong, fit, healthy body is an essential element in a happy, secure, psychologically healthy human being.

It has also become increasingly clear that a sturdy, energetic, well-nourished body is an important factor in having a comfortable and successful pregnancy and a healthy baby. The time to get your fitness level up and your eating habits in line is well before you start to try for pregnancy. What's ahead in this chapter is basically a summary of standard diet and exercise guidelines. You can get more detailed information on these subjects, and I encourage you to do so. But the point for you now is to start looking at this "old" information in a new way. A strong body adapts to the physical challenges of pregnancy more easily. A well-nourished body has the nutrient reserves for a developing fetus to draw on—calcium for building bones, for example, and iron to manufacture red blood cells.

Once you're pregnant, many of these basic rules will change. Later in the book I'll discuss diet and exercise guidelines to follow during pregnancy. For now, though, your goal should be to get—or stay— in shape, for your own health and the health of your future children.

FITNESS AND TRAINING BASICS

Picture a willowy ballerina in a graceful pirouette. Compare her to a lineman, mid-tackle; or a sinewy marathoner, striding steadily along. Each is, undeniably, an athlete, but it's hard to put a finger on any single common factor that links them together. Similarly, there is no one physical attribute in each of us to determine whether or not we are "fit." Instead, there are many components of physical fitness, each important in its own right. These include body composition (how much of the body is fat, how much is "lean" muscle, bone, water), flexibility (the degree to which muscles and joints let us bend, stretch, twist), and cardiovascular or aerobic efficiency (which measures the body's ability to extract oxygen from the air we breathe and speed it, via the blood, to every cell in the body, including working muscles).

Although each aspect of fitness is important to health, every woman should balance her exercise program to meet her own particular goals. Does she want to pare off excess fat? Be as lithe and flexible as a gymnast? Lower her risk of heart disease? Does she want to be able to run ten miles, lift her weight in steel plates, or prepare her body for pregnancy? Exercise is appropriate for every woman at every age; and it is particularly important for a woman contemplating pregnancy.

EXERCISE: THE BEST WAY TO LOSE WEIGHT

Being overweight at any age takes a health and psychological toll. But for a woman planning a pregnancy, there are two additional factors. First, the risks of toxemia and diabetes are increased in too-heavy pregnant women; and second, it's not a good idea to try to lose weight during gestation, since this would deprive a fetus of necessary nutrients. The best plan, then, is to try to get to a normal weight well beforehand.

It is very difficult to lose weight and keep it off by diet alone. This is because the body has a built-in diet detector. It senses and adjusts to caloric deprivation by lowering its metabolic rate. In other words, when you suddenly start to eat less, the body prepares to wait out a possible "famine" by slowing down in order to conserve fuel.

Another problem with eating much less to lose weight is that some of the weight loss will be from lean tissue—muscles, bones, organs. Lean tissue is not only vital to health, but also has a much higher metabolic rate than fat. Fat is basically stored fuel. It simply sits, stable, inert, waiting to be summoned out as a backup when other fuel sources are depleted. Lean tissue, on the other hand, is constantly being used, broken down, and repaired—processes that steadily consume calories.

If, instead of cutting calories to tip the fuel in/energy out balance in favor of weight loss, you increase the body's need for calories through exercise, the metabolic rate will remain stable, or even increase. And with a combination of your reducing food intake a bit and increasing activity as much as possible, the body doesn't receive a "slow down" alert; it heeds the signal to rev up, to be prepared to move. This strategy leads to slow but steady weight loss. The best types of exercise to add to your routine for weight loss are those that expend large amounts of calories. The choices include cycling, jogging, cross-country skiing, swimming, aerobic dance, and ordinary walking—activities that keep a large percentage of the body's muscles working over an extended period of time.

It is difficult to be patient when setting off on a weight-loss plan, but it is important to start up slowly. Think about joining a health club or exercise class, or setting up a regular workout schedule with someone of similar abilities. This is an excellent way to get through the early critical stages of an exercise plan—those first six months, when as many as 50 percent of women lose their resolve and drop out. It takes a long time to lose, say, twenty pounds. Perhaps six months, or even a year at the recommended rate of one or two pounds a week. But keep in mind that's only one year to shed, for *good*, weight that may have accumulated over a period of ten years or more.

FLEXIBILITY: THE BODY'S SHOCK ABSORBER

Joints and muscles can lose flexibility with age and lack of use, leaving the body stiff and injury-prone. But a good deal of mobility can be regained through correct stretching. Increase flexibility by moving each joint gently, without bouncing, to its current limit (the point at which you start to feel tension in the muscles), and then stretching just a bit beyond that point—but never so far that the tension becomes painful—for ten to thirty seconds.

Stretching to increase flexibility in any joint can loosen fingers stiff from gripping a pen for hours, or calves taut from a day of walking in high heels. Tightness in the back, trunk, and back-of-thigh muscles (hamstrings) is associated with back problems—which often worsen during pregnancy due to the added weight of the fetus. To test your flexibility in this area, sit on the floor and slowly reach for your toes.

Keep feet flexed so toes point to the ceiling. If there is a gap of more than two to three inches between your fingertips and your toes, your back muscles need to be stretched. Use this test as an exercise, holding the reach for ten to thirty seconds, or until you feel the tightness in your back and hamstrings ease.

AEROBIC CAPACITY: STAYING POWER

The rate at which you can keep walking, running, or pedaling a bike steadily for many minutes depends on your aerobic fitness—the body's ability to take in, transport, and use oxygen. The word "aerobic" means "with oxygen." If exercise is too intense, your body can't supply oxygen fast enough and it must make up the difference with less efficient anaerobic ("without oxygen") metabolism. A substance called "lactic acid" is then produced in the muscles. A large amount of lactic acid interferes with the muscles' smooth, efficient functioning and causes cramping pain. The idea is to reach a balance: to push the body only to the point at which lactic acid can be whisked away in the blood as quickly as it is produced. Then you can continue to exercise for long periods of time.

Of all the ways to measure fitness, aerobic capacity would probably top almost every doctor's list of the most important components. That's because, unlike flexibility or strength, the ability to endure in exercise—jog two miles, bike ten—is inextricably linked to some of the most important qualities of overall good health.

Coronary artery disease (impaired blood flow in the vessels that nourish the heart muscle itself) is a major cause of death in older women in the United States. But aerobic exercise, such as swimming, cycling, running, brisk walking, and cross-country skiing, can change a number of reactions in the body known to be risks for heart disease.

Although it isn't completely understood how this happens, regular aerobic exercise causes healthier patterns in the lipoproteins, which are the carriers of fat and cholesterol in the blood. Levels of the "bad" low-density lipoproteins, or LDL, tend to be lower in active people. Lowering too-high LDL levels has been shown to reduce the risk of heart attacks. "Good" high-density lipoproteins (HDL) protect against coronary artery disease. These particles seem to remove cholesterol from tissue, including the inner walls of the blood vessels. If left to collect on blood vessel walls, the cholesterol can form plaques that narrow the vessels, choke off the blood flow, and eventually block the tiny tubes completely, causing a heart attack—or a stroke if the vessel is in the brain. Very active women, such as runners, have been shown to have much higher HDL than their sedentary counterparts.

Before healthy changes can emerge in your HDL/LDL levels, aerobic workouts must be reasonably vigorous, such as running at least ten miles per week, kept up for six months or more.

In addition to blood fat changes, with aerobic fitness blood pressure tends to go down. The heart learns to do more work—pump more oxygen-rich blood each time it squeezes—with less effort. Aerobic training also markedly reduces how fast your heart beats at any given work rate. In fact, one way to tell you're getting more fit is to measure your resting pulse rate for a minute before you get out of bed in the morning. It will go down from an average of 80 beats or higher for an unfit woman to 60 or lower for a highly trained athlete.

WORKING OUT: HOW HARD? HOW LONG?

How can you tell how aerobically fit you are right now? One test is to measure the length of time it takes to cover (walking and/or running) a mile and a half of level ground. For a young woman, 11 minutes is excellent, 14 is average, and 17 is poor. To improve your score, you must "train" your body to improve its ability to use oxygen. Aerobic exercise at 50 to 85 percent of your body's maximum oxygen consumption has been shown to result in aerobic training. This corresponds to a heart rate of 60 to 90 percent of its maximum—a range called the "target heart rate" or "target zone." You can determine your target zone by subtracting your age from 220 (to get your age-adjusted maximum heart rate) and multiplying the result by 0.6 and 0.9. When you exercise, your heart rate per minute should be between those two numbers. (This is also the best range for burning as much fat as possible during exercise.)

Heart rate is measured easily by counting the pulse at your neck or wrist several times during a workout, to check the intensity of your exercise. Keep in mind that the heart rate target zone is a general guideline, not a rigid prescription. If you are very much out of shape you should exercise in the low end. Once you get into moderately good shape, it's okay to push yourself toward the higher end. (Some medical conditions and pregnancy will change the ideal target range for a particular person, at least temporarily.)

Another technique for measuring exercise intensity is known as "perceived exertion." This means just what it sounds like: Every work-out gives you an overall impression of where you are on a scale of very easy to very difficult. If you are young and healthy, and have no cardiovascular history, checking your heart rate may not be necessary every time you exercise. Once you've taken your pulse often enough—over a period of time—to know how being in the target heart rate *feels*, you will be able to keep the exercise at the correct level, some-where around "fairly hard."

The "sing-talk" method, although not very precise, can also be used to measure how hard you are working. If you cannot talk without gasping for breath while exercising, you have probably exceeded the target zone. If you can sing while exercising you are probably not pushing hard enough.

To achieve the training effect of improving oxygen uptake, aerobic workouts should last 15 to 30 minutes and be done three to five times a week. During the early phase of training, staying closer to 15 than 30 minutes and near the low end of your target zone will minimize the risks of injury as your body adapts to the increased activity.

Intensity, duration, and frequency of aerobic exercise should be increased gradually, one component at a time. A week or two at each new level will challenge the body to get stronger and more efficient without a stress overload. If, at any level, you feel you need more time there, don't hesitate to hold steady for a couple of weeks. You can even drop back a bit until your energy returns, or any recurrent ache or stiffness subsides. A day off between workouts is sensible at first to minimize stresses on the joints and ligaments. By gradually increasing your capacity you may be able to exercise daily. Varying your workouts will relieve parts of the body from continual stress and add a welcome change of pace for the mind as well. Try alternating days of brisk walking with biking or swimming, for example. Or switch from tennis to racquetball or running to skating, with the seasons.

Exercise should feel pleasurably tiring. If it is just pleasant you are probably not working hard enough. If it is only tiring you are working too hard. An hour after finishing your workout you should feel good, rested not exhausted.

A well-rounded exercise program should aim at improving flexibility and strength as well as aerobic capacity. Muscle-building calisthenics or weight lifting can be added to strengthen parts of the body neglected by your choice of aerobic exercise. This often includes the abdominal and upper body muscles. Strengthening exercises can be done before or after the aerobic phase of an exercise session; or you might alternate days of aerobic workouts with days of strength-training.

Whether done alone or as part of a longer workout, the aerobic segment must always begin with a warm-up and be followed by a cool-down. The warm-up, which increases circulation and prepares the body for harder work, can be simply five to ten minutes at a low intensity of whatever exercise you do: walking for a runner, leisurely laps for a swimmer, slow pedaling for a bike rider. The cool-down is the reverse. This slow segment after intense exercise keeps the blood from pooling in the extremities (where it's been concentrated to keep working muscles supplied with blood) and eases the body back to a lower level of activity. The cool-down should be continued until the pulse drops below 120 beats per minute, which usually takes about five to ten minutes. A few minutes of complete relaxation following each workout often reinforces the pleasure of exercise, and can make the transition to a high-energy lifestyle easier and more enjoyable.

Besides enhancing cardiovascular health, strength, and flexibility, and making weight control easier, there is one final advantage of regular exercise that should not be overlooked. Getting in shape can do an almost amazing amount of good for your psychological well-being. Regular exercisers feel better about themselves in general, and report finding relief from anger, tension, anxiety, and even mild to moderate depression through their chosen activities. A side benefit of exercise is that the feelings of mental and physical health it confers often encourage us to improve other habits as well—to eat better, sleep more regularly, cut down on smoking, alcohol, and drug use.

The goal of complete fitness is the strength and endurance to be able to do what you want your body to do—walk to the store, play three sets of tennis, carry a baby with grace and energy to spare—combined with the flexibility to give with a sudden twist without snapping—the way tree limbs sway in the wind.

HEALTHY EATING

"You are what you eat." How many times have you heard this? But it's not just a clever play on words; it's quite literally true. Food is the stuff our bodies are made of. It is what every tissue is composed of and sustained by. It is the fuel that every organ and body process— breathing, digestion, circulation—runs on. And when a woman is pregnant, what she eats becomes the stuff the developing fetus is made of, as well.

Most of us, however, don't give much thought to what our bodies physically need when we sit down to a meal, or grab a handful of potato chips, or opt for a dinner of Chinese or Mexican. That's because food, in our society, is much more than simply fuel. It has strong psychological and social implications as well. And there's nothing wrong with that.

What is important, though, is to increase our awareness of food's critical role in our well-being and incorporate that knowledge into our daily eating decisions. You can, for example, get all the essential nutrients from a vegetarian diet as well as from an all-American meat- and-potatoes one. But to do this, you need to know just a few nutrition basics.

In essence, when we talk about the food the body cannot survive without, we're talking about what nutritionists dub "essential nu- trients"—those substances the body must get in food to keep itself healthy because it can't make them itself. There are six main categories of essential nutrients: carbohydrates, fats, protein, minerals, vitamins, and water.

CARBOHYDRATES: THE FUEL WE RUN ON

As recently as a couple of years ago, carbohydrates were seen as the villain, the food to be avoided if you wanted to stay, or get, thin. In fact, carbohydrates are the main fuel the body runs on, and getting more, not less, is starting to be acknowledged as one of the real keys to attaining healthy slimness.

The reason carbohydrates got their bad rep probably comes from the fact that there are two types in most people's diets: simple and complex. The chemical building block of all carbohydrates is one or more monosaccharides (you've heard of some of them—glucose, fruc- tose, galactose), and the further you get from these basic chunks the more complex a carbohydrate is. The body must break any carbohy- drate down into its simple sugars to use the energy stored in it. Sucrose, or table sugar, is made of two monosaccharides—glucose and fruc- tose—so it must be, basically, just split in two before the body can use it. Other carbohydrates must go through an elaborate breaking-down process, and some, such as fiber, cannot be broken down at all in our digestive tracts.

Simple sugars, then, aren't inherently bad; they're very easy for the body to use, and they don't take up much space. In other words, you can eat lots of them without feeling full. Unfortunately, the body doesn't excrete any extra sugars you may eat beyond your calorie burn-off needs. It simply puts them into storage, as fat. Complex carbohydrates, on the other hand, are bulky, take your body more energy to digest (which, by the way, means simply to break them down into a body-usable form), and make you feel full and satisfied quickly. Because of this, it's harder to eat more than your physical energy needs require. The bottom line: On a high-complex-carbohydrate diet, you're less likely to get fat.

A high-complex-carbohydrate, low-simple-carbohydrate diet has also been linked to a lower risk of certain kinds of cancer, heart disease, diabetes, even dental cavities! Part of the "complexity" of complex carbs, too, is that they come packaged with many of the vitamins and minerals essential to keeping your body functioning smoothly. So they're not only a "diet miracle," they're a "vitamin pill," too!

Complex carbohydrates are basically found in plant foods, including fruits and vegetables, beans and grains (especially unrefined grains like whole wheat, bran, oats, buckwheat). Ideally, you want half or more of your total calorie intake to come from these food sources.

FAT: NOT JUST A DIRTY WORD

Just the word "fat" makes people cringe. The basic reason for this is that, gram for gram, fat packs twice the calories of carbohydrates or protein. While that makes fats extremely efficient at their job—storage of energy in case of a cut-off in the food supply—it also makes them double trouble in societies of high living standards, like ours, where an overabundance of food is likely to be a health problem.

Fat is not *just* inert storage; it is also essential to the body. It is a constituent of cell walls, helping the cell regulate the intake and excretion of nutrients. The fat beneath the skin—so-called subcutaneous fat—is an insulator, protecting the body from changes in temperature in the outside world. Of course, too much subcutaneous fat, in the form of rolls and lumps, isn't necessary for temperature control (and may in fact impede it) and poses very real health risks and psychological problems.

Most of the fat we get in our diets is in straight, visible fat form: the oils we put in salad dressings, the butter on the baked potatoes and vegetables, the shortening mixed into cookies and cakes and breads. Another large percentage comes as an "extra" in animal foods. This includes both the visible fat wrapped around a juicy steak and the bits of white "marbling" running through the meat. Meats vary tremendously in the amount of fat they contain. Since I used beef as an example, you might guess that a high percentage of the calories in a piece of steak come from fat. The same is true of pork. A slice of chicken or turkey has much less fat, as does fish. A much smaller percentage of fats in our diet come from plant foods—vegetables and grains and nuts; but when cutting down on fat is of major concern, these sources can be important to consider.

Many people get up to, and even more than, half their calories from fat. A much healthier proportion would be 20 to 30 percent; but you'd be surprised how hard it is to get your diet down to that figure. Nobody's saying every salad should be eaten without dressing, or every potato without a dollop of sour cream. But any nutritionist would be quick to point out that the whole tasty, filling potato may have about 100 calories, while just one tablespoon of butter melted on top of it has an equal amount. And the salad dressing almost always has more calories than the salad itself.

Your *total* fat intake isn't the only issue. The *type of fat* matters too. Put very simply, fats that are solid at room temperature—butter and the fats in meats, for example—tend to increase your risk of heart-attack-causing fatty deposits building up inside blood vessels. Fats that are liquid at room temperature—most oils—tend not to. Some experts recommend that the solid fats (called saturated fats) be limited to no more than 15 percent of your total calories.

PROTEIN: THE BODY'S BUILDING BLOCKS

Probably nobody needs to try to convince you that protein is of critical importance as a nutrient. It is a component of every living cell. All the enzymes that regulate metabolic processes in the body are proteins; and many hormones are either proteins or protein derivatives.

The basic blocks from which all proteins are built are amino acids. And how useful a food protein will be to the body comes down to how well that food's amino acids match up with the balance that humans need. Almost all animal proteins—including those in meat, milk, and eggs—are "complete," meaning they have all the amino acids the body needs. Since it's simple to get the right balance with these foods, we have come to rely on them for most of our protein. The drawbacks are that these tend to be economically expensive sources of protein and that the protein often comes packaged with a lot of fat.

The other source of amino acids is plant foods. They usually are much less expensive and much lower in fat. However, you have to work a bit to make sure you're getting the right balance of amino acids here, since plant foods are all "incomplete proteins"—meaning they're missing one or more essential amino acids. An easy way to "complete" plant protein is to add just a bit of a complete protein to it. A little ground beef in your spaghetti sauce, a handful of cheese on your vegetable or macaroni casserole, a splash of milk on your cereal all allow your body to use much more of the vegetable protein than it could otherwise. A little harder, but something vegetarians do as a matter of course, is to learn some combinations of plant foods that, eaten together, add up to the complete protein your body can use. The classic Mexican rice and beans combo is one example; peanut butter on whole wheat bread is another.

Roughly speaking, 20 percent or less of your daily calorie intake should be protein. Most Americans eat much more protein than they need. Men between the ages of twenty-three and fifty need about 50–60 grams a day. Women the same age need about 10 grams less. A pregnant woman needs about 30 grams more a day, and a nursing mother 20 extra.

Minerals and Vitamins

Compared with the sheer bulk of the food elements, the tiny bits of vitamins and minerals we need for health may make them easy to overlook. And because we normally get most of the vitamins and minerals we need in the foods we eat, we may be even more tempted to take them for granted. That would be a serious mistake.

What do minerals do? For one thing, they maintain the correct acid/base balance in the body for chemical reactions to occur. Scores of chemical reactions go on constantly in every cell; most often they need just the right environment to do so. All the energy in the form of glucose or fats and all the building blocks in the form of amino acids can be right there, but if your body can't use them, they're worthless. Minerals are also sometimes parts of essential body compounds: Bone wouldn't be bone without calcium; hemoglobin, the oxygen-carrying part of the blood, needs iron to do its critical job. Minerals are necessary for muscles to be able to contract, and for nerves to send their messages speeding along their length. And much, much more.

There are as many as sixty different minerals in the human body; over twenty have been clearly identified as having essential roles in maintaining life, growth, and the ability to reproduce. The list of essential minerals keeps growing as nutritionists learn more and more about the wondrously complex workings of the body. That's one reason experts recommend eating a wide variety of foods—some may contain minerals our bodies need that we haven't discovered yet—instead of relying on mineral supplements.

Minerals are classified as "macronutrients"—meaning they're needed in relatively large amounts—or "micronutrients" if only tiny amounts are necessary for the body to carry out its daily duties. Examples of macronutrients include calcium, potassium, sodium, and magnesium. Micronutrients include iron, zinc, iodine, nickel, and tin.

Vitamins, like minerals, are tiny bits of substances we can't live without. That said, I would also like to point out that alone they can't keep us alive. No vitamin and mineral tablet, no matter how balanced and complete, can keep your body going without food. The only reason such supplements were designed in the first place is that some of us find it difficult to eat a large enough variety of foods to ensure that all the needed vitamins and minerals are included along with the carbohydrates, fats, and proteins. And that's fine. But just remember, these pills are supplements to good nutrition, not good nutrition itself.

Vitamins come in two broad groups. There are four fat-soluble vitamins—A, D, E, and K. And there are eleven water-soluble vitamins—ten of which are known as the "B complex," which includes thiamin, riboflavin, folacin, and biotin, and the last of which is vitamin C. One of the major differences between the two groups is that the body can store fat-soluble vitamins if you eat more than you need; so that you don't have to get them every day. Water-soluble vitamins are excreted from the body if they're eaten in excess, so you have to keep taking in new supplies every day. Sometimes too much of certain vitamins can cause as many problems as too little—another reason taking supplements without a clear purpose is discouraged by nutrition experts.

WATER: MOST VITAL OF ALL

No single nutrient could possibly be said to have a more central role in life than water. Although the exact proportion varies, more than half of the average adult's body is water. No cell can live without it.

Water is the transporter of vital nutrients from one part of the body to another. Sugars for energy, amino acids for cell-building, vitamins, minerals, and hormones all travel dissolved in the water of the bloodstream and lymphatic systems. It is a necessary part of chemical reactions, such as the breaking down of complex nutrients into smaller units the body can use. It helps to regulate body temperature.

The body loses water constantly, in urine, through sweating (which you do all the time, whether you notice it or not), as you breathe, and occasionally through vomiting and diarrhea. Obviously, then, it is of major importance to keep your body supplied with enough water, to keep it, as physicians say, well-hydrated. As a general rule, it's suggested that the average adult, lounging about in 72° weather, needs about 22 milliliters of water per kilogram (2.2 pounds) of body weight (40 ounces for a 120-pound person). At 100°, you'd need about 38 milliliters of water per kilogram (70 ounces for a 120-pound person), or about a quart more than at 72°. Usually about two-thirds of this comes from drinks, the rest from solid foods.

ENERGY BALANCE: CALORIES IN, CALORIES OUT

The last nutrition topic I'll discuss is one I touched on earlier in the exercise section: the total energy balance that tips your scale in the direction of weight gain or weight loss, or just keeps your weight holding steady.

If you want to gain weight, you have to take in more calories and burn up fewer; if you want to lose weight, you have to take in fewer and burn up more. This is easy to say and very difficult to translate into practice. Since we eat to satisfy much more than our body's simple need for nutrients, cutting down on eating is, in itself, no simple task. It's also very difficult to determine exactly how many calories your body needs. There's a certain baseline requirement you use just by being alive. This "basal metabolic rate" (BMR) includes calories that keep blood coursing through your veins, your lungs pulling in fresh oxygen and getting rid of carbon dioxide, your brain working, and allows other processes that don't stop when you're asleep or quietly reading a book. Added to the BMR is any caloric expenditure for movement—from walking up a flight of stairs to running a 26-mile marathon, and everything in between.

But even that doesn't hint at the complexity of the calorie in/calorie out balance. You've probably seen charts and tables on how many calories it takes to walk a mile or swim a few laps in a pool, or do a little light gardening. (I've even included a few in this book for reference.) But these numbers are just rough approximations. Your exact needs vary depending on many factors. How in shape are you? What's your body's proportion of fat to lean? How old are you? How hot is it outside? How energetically do you do the activity in question, and how good at doing it are you? It's easy to say a pound of fat stores about 3,500 calories, but a very different thing to get your body to actually use up that much-despised pound of fat.

The only way to know what will work for your body right now is to cut back a bit on the calories you eat and see what happens. As I hope

TABLE 1

COMPARATIVE TABLE OF CALORIES IN/CALORIES OUT

| | | MINUTES OF ACTIVITY REQUIRED TO BURN UP CALORIES | | |
FOOD	CALORIES	IN WALKING	IN BICYCLING	IN RUNNING
Apple	100	19	12	5
Beer (1 glass)	115	22	14	6
Raw carrot	42	8	5	2
Cottage cheese (1 tbsp.)	27	5	3	1
Ice cream (1/6 pint)	193	37	24	10
Pizza (1 slice)	180	35	22	9
Hamburger	350	67	42	18
Orange	68	13	8	4

SOURCE: Modified from *For Women of All Ages*, S. H. Cherry, M.D., Macmillan Co., New York.

I've impressed upon you so far, what you eat is so critical to your health and well-being, it's obviously playing with fire either to drastically cut down the total number of calories you eat or simply to axe any one food group from your eat-list. Instead, try to eat just a little bit less—a mouthful here and there can make an astonishing difference over a week, a month, several years—of pretty much what you've been eating now. Of course, if your diet is too high in fats or simple carbohydrates you should try to bring them into healthier balance as well, but as far as just straight energy balance goes, it's the total number of calories that counts.

A healthy weight loss will go no faster than two pounds a week, average. Faster than that, and you're probably disturbing the body's water balance and excreting water rather than fat, and you won't be able to sustain that rate of loss anyway. Another number that's useful to start with is 500. If you were to eat 500 fewer calories per day, and increase the amount of exercise you get by another 500 calories (as closely as you can figure, of course), you should be working at a deficit of 1,000 calories a day. One thousand times seven is 7,000, which is exactly two pounds' worth of calories per week.

As soon as you start to think about getting pregnant, you should first plan to get your body in shape. If you're not sure what a healthy weight is for you, ask your doctor. Then you can work backward from your planned conception time, following the two-pounds-a-week rule. Give yourself some leeway, too, so the process can be as relaxed and gradual—and enjoyable—as possible. By the time you're ready to get pregnant you may just be in better shape than ever before.

4

Contraception

The choice in contraception is something every woman, and every couple, has to grapple with. As soon as the decision is made to have sex, some kind of decision about birth control also has to be made. And this isn't a one-time choice, either: The "right" contraceptive varies from couple to couple, and it changes for any one woman during her sexually active years. A young woman who may still be seeking a long-term partner has very different needs from a newly married couple looking forward to starting a family. And the woman who plans to establish her career before having children faces yet another set of options. A birth control method must also be considered from an aesthetic viewpoint: It must be as pleasant to use as possible—or it *won't* be used consistently and correctly. And using any method carefully, every time, is the key to effectiveness.

Another concern is constant for each woman who still sees childbearing in her future: She needs a method that is as safe as possible, as effective as possible, that will not jeopardize her ability to have children when she decides to do so. Most readers of this book will fall into that category. A woman who has completed her family has a somewhat different contraceptive outlook. She and her partner may even, for example, want to consider one of the forms of sterilization.

Unfortunately, there is no perfect method of birth control. Every technique has its side effects, drawbacks, or limitations as well as its advantages. Some methods—the IUD, for example—may be distinctly hazardous to women who want no risks to their subsequent fertility. Others, such as the diaphragm, may be extremely safe, but the tradeoff is a slightly higher pregnancy rate. Together, you and your physician can make the best decision about the method that works for you right now without causing problems in the future. Try to be open and clear about your needs, likes, and dislikes, and take the time to do a little homework about various methods so you can talk to your doctor about them.

Most reversible methods of contraception fall into one of three general categories: a barrier method, hormonal method, or intrauterine device method. Other, less effective techniques, such as withdrawal and rhythm, will be discussed. The permanent birth control option, sterilization for either the man or woman, will not be covered since it is not yet an issue for the couples for whom I wrote this book: those who are concerned with preserving their fertility.

BARRIER METHODS OF CONTRACEPTION

The barrier methods—so called because they work by physically keeping sperm from egg—are among the oldest forms of birth control. In Egypt, medicated vaginal inserts are mentioned as early as 1500 B.C. Condoms also have been used since ancient times. The original models were fashioned from the intestines of animals. Modern-day barrier contraceptives began to appear toward the end of the nineteenth century: primitive diaphragms, cervical caps, and condoms. For many years, these were the only birth control methods available.

In addition to preventing pregnancy, the barrier methods also provide a bonus to women concerned about their future reproductive health. It appears that spermicidal jellies, creams, and foams may inhibit the growth of some of the organisms associated with sexually transmittable diseases—gonorrhea, syphilis, trichomonas, and, perhaps, even herpes. These infections are known to be able to cause infertility.

There has been a recent increase in the use of barrier methods because of their safety and the availability of some of them without a doctor's prescription. They also appeal to women who are postponing the start of their families until their late twenties or thirties, and are concerned about the effects of exposure to the Pill's hormones or the IUD's risk of infection. Barrier methods are also particularly attractive to women who have sex infrequently or sporadically. "I don't have to take a pill every day or live with a foreign object in my uterus. I just use birth control when I need it" was how a young single woman put it. The availability of safe, legal, early abortion also allows some women to accept the tradeoff involved in using methods that are absolutely safe but less than 100 percent effective.

The fact that barrier methods must be used every time you have sex, however, deters many potential users. Couples may find it inconvenient and distracting to pause in their lovemaking or to prepare in advance for sex. Some women find the spermicides too greasy and messy ("My diaphragm is like a wild thing, skidding out of my hands and boinging all over!") or are disturbed by the sensation of heat and itching that they sometimes produce; and men complain that "it just doesn't *feel* the same" with condoms. The attitude of the man is also important for the use of some vaginal spermicides, since his cooperation will be necessary in waiting the proper length of time for a suppository to melt or foam.

□ *The diaphragm* was known prior to the introduction of the Pill and the intrauterine device (IUD) as the most frequently used form of contraception in the United States. Diaphragms are shallow rubber cups with flexible metal rims that fold or bend for insertion, then pop open and slide into place, covering the cervix. They have two roles: first, to provide a physical barrier that keeps sperm from getting into the cervix; and, second, to hold spermicidal gels and creams that increase the method's effectiveness by immobilizing sperm that try to sneak in around the rim. There are many types of diaphragm currently in use, but the design of all of them is basically similar. The effectiveness of the diaphragm at preventing pregnancy depends on two factors: getting the right type and fit, and using it correctly and consistently. The correct type and size of diaphragm depends on your pelvic anatomy and vaginal tone. Since only your doctor can determine this for you, diaphragms cannot be obtained without a prescription. The vagina expands during sexual excitement, so the largest diaphragm that fits and is comfortable is the one that should be used. If it is too small, it may slip out of place. If it is too big, it may rotate and not cover the cervix. Therefore, it is essential that an experienced person fit a diaphragm. Childbirth may change the size and shape of the vagina, so a new fitting is required after pregnancy before sex is resumed. Some physicians also recommend a new fitting if a weight change of fifteen to twenty pounds occurs.

You should be taught how to use and care for the diaphragm when you are first fitted for it. The diaphragm must be inserted before sexual intercourse. "If I have to stop and go to the bathroom to put my diaphragm in, I don't even *want* to have sex anymore once I'm done!" one woman complained. So she and her partner learned to incorporate insertion into their foreplay. Other couples also see stopping to do this an interruption and prefer to insert the diaphragm up to an hour or so before sex begins. Before it is slipped into place, a teaspoonful (or applicatorful) of jelly or cream is placed inside the dome, which will cover the cervix, and a little bit more is spread around the entire rim (Figure 7). After insertion the woman, or her partner, should slide a finger into the vagina to check that the diaphragm is, in fact, covering the cervix. Neither you nor your partner should be able to feel the diaphragm, if it is correctly in place. A woman can walk around, go to work, or bathe with it in place; and a man should not be able to feel it ("run into it") during sex. Let your doctor know if this is not the case.

The diaphragm is left in place for at least six, preferably eight, hours after the last time you have sex. If intercourse should occur again while the diaphragm is in place, you should first insert another applicatorful

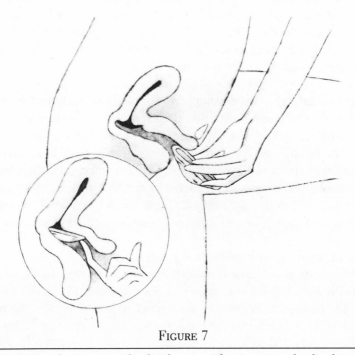

FIGURE 7

Technique for inserting the diaphragm. After inserting the diaphragm, a finger is inserted into the vagina to check for placement over the cervix.

of spermicidal jelly or cream *without removing the diaphragm*. (A diaphragm can be used during menstruation, but should be removed as soon as possible after the required time because of the slight risk of Toxic Shock Syndrome.)

Six or more hours after the last time you have sex, the diaphragm can be carefully removed. (Although they are quite sturdy, a fingernail can tear them.) The diaphragm is then washed with warm water and a mild soap and dried. Some women dust it lightly with cornstarch before storing. (Talcum powder should *not* be used because of its possible relationship to cancer of the ovary.) Before storing, it should be inspected for small holes or rips—they are easiest to spot if you hold it up to the light. With careful handling, a diaphragm generally lasts about two years.

When the diaphragm fails, it may be due to a poor fit, a hole or tear in the device, failure to add spermicide for repeated sex, taking it out too soon, or failure to use it at all. Theoretically—if it is used correctly every time—its effectiveness should be about 98 percent: If 100 women used it for a year, 2 would get pregnant. However, since we are human and occasionally impatient, careless, or forgetful, its actual effectiveness is quite a bit less—about 92 percent. The cost of the diaphragm is about $10, plus the cost of spermicide, plus the cost of the initial visit to your physician.

☐ *The cervical cap* was developed in the mid-nineteenth century by a German gynecologist. A thimble-shaped rubber device that was fitted over a woman's cervix, the cap was custom-made from a wax impression of each user's cervix. Although cervical caps have been used in Europe, they never achieved widespread acceptance. Their use today is minimal because they are much more difficult to insert properly and remove than the diaphragm. "You need the fingers of a spider monkey to get it in and out!" a woman who tried to use one informed me.

The cervical cap is smaller than a diaphragm, fits directly over the cervix (instead of blocking the entire upper part of the vaginal canal, as a diaphragm does), and is made out of a more rigid plastic or rubber. Recently the cap has achieved a resurgence in popularity and interest, since new research efforts have made them easier to insert and remove, and they can be left in place for longer time periods. Currently, however, the cap is used much like the diaphragm, being filled with spermicide prior to use, and left in six to eight hours following intercourse. The cervical cap is not approved for general use in this country by the Food and Drug Administration (FDA) for two reasons. One is that the pregnancy rates associated with its use are high. Second, it is irritating to the cervix. More research and development is needed.

☐ *Vaginal spermicides* are sperm-killing (spermicidal) agents placed inside the vagina before sex, a very old method of birth control. Over the ages many different preparations have been used. Currently, vaginal spermicides come in five general forms: jellies, creams, suppositories, aerosol foams, and foaming tablets. While the form may vary, basically they all contain the same spermicide, nonoxynol-9.

It is essential that spermicides be used prior to each act of intercourse and in the proper manner. They must be placed where they will cover the cervix completely. If intercourse does not take place within one hour, a new application should be used. If foaming tablets or suppositories, which melt, are used, you must wait the stated length of time after putting them in before you can have sex. Douching should be avoided for at least six hours after the last act of intercourse, since it can take that long for all the sperm to be killed.

Spermicides have the advantage of being available over the counter, without a prescription, but the tradeoff is their relatively high failure rate: as much as 10 percent.

☐ *The sponge* is a new method of birth control. It is a synthetic sponge saturated with the same spermicide, nonoxynol-9, used in other vaginal contraceptives. Before the sponge is inserted, it is moistened with water to activate the spermicide; then it is pushed deep into the vagina until it covers the cervix. It is similar to the diaphragm in that it must remain in place for six to eight hours after sex, but you don't have to add spermicide if you have sex more than once. (Its proponents suggest that the sponge can be left in place for up to twenty-four hours, even with repeated sex during that time.)

The data on the sponge are still incomplete. It is reported to be almost as effective as a diaphragm. However, my recent experience with this method suggests a higher contraceptive failure rate than previously reported (perhaps due to incorrect use). There have been a few regrettable cases of Toxic Shock Syndrome with the sponge, although this does not appear to be a major problem at this time. One fairly significant advantage, on the other hand, is that "it's so much less messy than smearing on diaphragm goop all the time," as one woman put it. It's also available over the counter, is easily disposable, costs about a dollar each, and comes in packages of three, six, or twelve.

☐ *Condoms* are the only major, established form of male barrier contraception used today. The newest condoms, usually made of latex, are greatly improved—thinner, and often prelubricated. It is the method most often used in Japan, Sweden, and the United Kingdom and is, in fact, the most widely used form of contraception in the world.

Though the condom's theoretical effectiveness is an impressive 97 to 98 percent, its actual in-use effectiveness varies from population to population. Most failures are due to ripping or tearing. Less common reasons include putting the penis in the vagina before slipping on the condom, failure to unroll the condom completely on the shaft of the penis, and failure to leave enough space for the ejaculate at the tip of the condom. Add a vaginal spermicide to condom use and the effectiveness shoots up to a remarkable 99 percent! The condom-plus-spermicide is, in fact, probably the most underrated form of birth control in the United States today. "I always pictured adolescent boys fumbling around in backseats of cars when I thought of condoms," a twenty-eight-year-old said to me. "But they're really a responsible, effective method that's right for my husband and me until we want kids."

In addition to being a highly effective contraceptive, condoms are a very good protection against many types of sexually transmitted diseases. They are inexpensive and available over the counter, without prescription. The major drawback for women, however, is that they must rely upon their male partner to use this method. Many males are reluctant to do so.

BIRTH CONTROL PILLS

One of the great scientific advances of the past thirty years was the development of the highly effective, easy-to-use oral contraceptive. More than 100 million women have used the birth control pill; perhaps over 10 million women are currently taking it in this country.

The idea of an oral contraceptive arose from the fact that pregnancy temporarily shuts down the process of ovulation. In the early 1950s, female sex hormones were first administered to mimic a pregnancy hormonally and block ovulation, and Pill development was off and running. In 1960 the U.S. Food and Drug Administration (FDA) authorized the marketing of Enovid, the first birth control pill. Since then, massive inputs of time, effort, and money have gone into the refinement of the oral contraceptive.

Taken as directed (twenty-one days on, seven days off—during which bleeding occurs), the combination estrogen/progesterone Pill is virtually 100 percent effective from the very first cycle. In some ways it is close to the ideal method: It is quite safe, easily reversible, and as simple to take as swallowing a tiny tablet once a day. "But aren't they dangerous?" I'm often asked. Yes, there are potential side effects, which in a very small number of cases can be serious. And it was these side effects that gave the Pill a largely unwarranted dangerous reputation a few years back, a setback from which this method is only now starting to recover. In the lower hormone doses used today, the benefits of oral contraceptives far outweigh their potential dangers for most women, especially healthy, young nonsmokers.

There are two major types of birth control pills: "combination" pills with estrogen and progesterone, and "mini" pills with progesterone alone. The protection against pregnancy with progesterone-alone pills is not as high as with the combined pill, and there is frequently irregular menstrual bleeding. For these reasons, the progesterone pills are used by only a small percentage of women who have specific medical reasons for not taking estrogen.

The effectiveness of oral contraceptives was for many years attributed solely to their ability to stop ovulation. However, eventually it was discovered that they also act on the cervix, producing a thick mucus barrier that sperm have trouble penetrating.

The amount of hormones in the Pill has been gradually reduced over the years, which has made side effects less common without decreasing effectiveness. The pills with the lowest dose of estrogen (35 to 50 micrograms) are currently recommended for most women to start with. Earlier pills had twice this hormone dose, or even more.

Every woman who takes birth control pills needs a thorough gynecologic checkup, Pap smear, and breast examination. A complete medical history should also be taken before the Pill is prescribed. Women with a history of blood clots, heart disease, cancer of the breast, high blood pressure, diabetes, epilepsy, migraine headaches, kidney disease, uterine fibroids, depression, or abnormal vaginal bleeding may not be able to take the Pill safely.

Women over thirty who smoke a pack or more of cigarettes a day and who take birth control pills are at greater risk of developing heart disease and strokes. Although the risks versus the benefits must be evaluated on an individual basis, most physicians are very cautious in prescribing the Pill for these women.

When pregnancy is desired, the contraceptive action of the Pill is easily reversed: You simply finish one Pill packet and do not start the next. Most physicians recommend the use of a barrier method for one to three months before attempting pregnancy, so a woman's natural menstrual cycle reestablishes itself; there is a slightly higher miscarriage rate in women who conceive in the first three months. Except for that, the pregnancy rate after using the birth control pills is exactly the same as that in women who have never taken it: 90 percent will become pregnant within one year. Women who have had irregular menstrual cycles may not immediately return to regular ovulation after stopping oral contraceptives. However, these women can be treated by other methods.

Questions have been raised occasionally about possible links between use of oral contraceptives and certain kinds of cancer. However, there is no evidence to date to support a cause-and-effect relationship. In fact, the opposite may well be true. Some studies have shown a decreased frequency of breast and ovarian cancer in women who have taken birth control pills.

Although a lot of attention has been given to potential adverse effects of oral contraceptives, they actually have certain beneficial side effects in addition to their contraceptive efficacy. Many women report a decrease of both pain in their periods and of premenstrual tension because the Pill inhibits ovulation. Women who have excessive bleeding with their periods find their flow decreases. Acne may improve. The Pill also produces regular cycles, which gives some women a sense of well-being and good health.

That's not to say that there are no side effects. There are. Some are more common than others, and some much more serious than others. Nausea is one minor side effect that is common during the first couple of cycles. It can usually be avoided by changing the time of day the Pill is taken, from morning to midday or before going to bed, for example. Breast enlargement is also common during the early cycles. Fluid retention is a problem for some, which can show up as bloating or swelling of the legs. There may be an increase in vaginal discharge. A patchy discoloration in facial pigmentation, called "chloasma," sometimes called "liver spots," can occur, especially when the Pill user is exposed to sunlight. (This condition is not always completely reversible when the Pill is stopped.) Some women experience mild mood changes, including depression, as well as increased appetite and weight gain. Recurrent vaginal infections—especially yeast infections—are more common among women on the Pill. In addition, certain drugs (such as tetracycline, ampicillin, and barbiturates) have been known to reduce the effectiveness of the Pill; and your doctor may suggest using a backup barrier method while you're taking them.

Occasionally, there will be no bleeding period during the seven days "off" the Pill. This is usually due to the fact that low-estrogen pills do not stimulate adequate buildup of the endometrium during the three weeks "on." This is generally not of concern since the bleeding is not a true period (there is no ovulation) but an artificial one, anyway. However, if you or your physician feels more comfortable if you have some "withdrawal bleeding," as it is known, the dose of estrogen in the tablet may be raised slightly. If you do not mind not bleeding, and don't constantly worry that no period is a sign of pregnancy, then the current medication schedule is continued. Even though the chances of pregnancy are minute if the Pill has been taken as directed, if the lack of bleeding persists, it will be necessary to do a pregnancy test.

Breakthrough bleeding, or bleeding in mid-pill-cycle, is due to an insufficient amount of estrogen in the birth control pill. Some physicians treat breakthrough bleeding by telling a woman to double up on pills the day the bleeding begins. Others prefer to have the woman finish the cycle as usual, then increase the estrogen a bit in the next cycle, by switching pill formulations. Breakthrough bleeding is also more common if tablets are missed.

When a woman forgets to take one or more tablets she should be aware that, for the rest of that cycle, effectiveness drops and a pregnancy could occur. Although pills should be continued until the end of the cycle, another method of birth control, such as a barrier method, should be used as a backup.

The serious complication associated with Pill use is an increased risk of blood clots in veins, which could possibly lead to an embolus— or traveling blood clot—in the lungs. It is not necessary to stop the use of oral contraceptives for a rest period periodically. This may result in an unwanted pregnancy, and there is no evidence that this will in any way reduce the side effects. Leg pains, chest pains, headaches, blurred vision, and shortness of breath may be danger symptoms while taking the Pill. These symptoms should be reported to your physician immediately.

Although oral contraceptives do not completely meet all criteria for the ideal contraceptive, the Pill often comes closer to this than any other technique. The birth control pill has proven to be safer than was thought for some time (especially in lower hormone doses and particularly in healthy women), and the risk of pregnancy is really negligible when it is taken correctly. As more women change to the lower-dose preparations the overall number of side effects may come down even more. Knowing this, and talking to your doctor about any worries, may help to reduce anxiety about taking the Pill, which is probably the ideal method for many women.

☐ *The "Morning-After" Pill*   For many years it has been known that giving a woman estrogen after intercourse at a fertile time may protect against pregnancy. To work, it must be taken not more than 48 hours after intercourse. Sooner is better, as there is a higher degree of effectiveness when used early.

Side effects are very common with the "morning-after" pill. Nausea and vomiting, abnormal bleeding, and breast tenderness frequently occur, since the dose of estrogen is quite high. Because of these and other potential side effects, the morning-after pill should never be considered an ongoing contraceptive method. It should be used only in emergencies.

If the morning-after pill doesn't work for one reason or another and a pregnancy should occur, an abortion should be considered. The occurrence of fetal abnormalities due to the use of estrogens during pregnancy has been well documented (for example, the DES tragedy, which is explained in Chapter 13, "Environmental Hazards to Pregnancy").

INTRAUTERINE DEVICES: IUDs

For over 2,000 years it has been known that a foreign object or device placed in the uterus could prevent pregnancy. Ancient Arabs and Turks placed pebbles in the uteruses of their female camels in order to protect them against pregnancy during their long journeys across the desert.

Over the years intrauterine devices were designed from various types of materials, but they gained little acceptance until the late 1950s and the discovery of biologically inert plastics—materials that did not interact with the body. Plastics were first used in "coil" and "loop" types of IUDs. Most of these early devices, including the bow, the Dalkon shield, and numerous others, have since been discontinued because of problems with insertion, removal, or infection.

In 1968 the FDA concluded that the IUD was a generally safe and effective form of birth control. The IUD has advantages for some women and, in many ways, may approach the ideal in contraceptives. It is inexpensive and is usually easy to insert with minimal complications. There is no interference with sexual intercourse at all. Side effects and pregnancy rates are quite low. (The IUD is about 98 percent effective.) Once contraception is no longer desired, the removal of an IUD is normally simple and uncomplicated. Pregnancy rates after IUD removal are normal.

IUDs are usually recommended for older women, for two main reasons: First, women face an increased risk with a birth control pill as they get older; second, the main drawback to the IUD is the risk of pelvic infection, and pelvic infection associated with IUD use may lead to sterility. This is an extremely important decision for women who have delayed childbearing or who still wish to have another pregnancy. Therefore, I advise my patients of this risk, and many decide to reserve the use of the IUD until they have completed their families.

There are basically three types of IUD in use today. The first, and older, kind consists of an inert plastic in varying shapes, which can remain in the uterus indefinitely. The second, a more recent development, consists of a segment of plastic to which a piece of copper has been attached. These so-called copper IUDs produce more effective contraception (a lower pregnancy rate). However, since the copper dissolves over time, this type of device must be periodically replaced, generally every three years.

More recently, a third type of IUD has been developed. It consists of an inert plastic to which the hormone progesterone has been added. The hormone is slowly released to enhance the contraceptive effect. This type of device must be replaced every year. If you are considering an IUD, ask your physician which type may be best for you. Recently two IUD manufacturers have stopped marketing their products in the United States (the Copper-T, Copper-7 and the Lippe's Loop). Their reasons seem to be legal rather than medical; the FDA still approves of these two products. If you are wearing one of these types of IUD there is no reason to remove it now unless pregnancy is desired. As I write this, only the progesterone-type IUD is available in the United States. The other types are available worldwide.

There are many theories as to how the IUD works, but none has been proven conclusively. It has been suggested that the IUD somehow changes the lining of the uterus so that the fertilized ovum cannot implant, or that it produces a muscle imbalance between the Fallopian tube and the uterus, hindering fertilization. Some alteration of the chemical environment of the uterus may also occur with the noninert IUDs, which prevents fertilization and/or implantation.

An IUD is inserted by your physician in the office, sometimes using a local anaesthetic. Insertion is timed to coincide with or follow a menstrual period or, less frequently, immediately following an abortion or at a postpartum visit. At this time a woman can be sure she is not pregnant, and the cervix is often slightly more open, as well. Some women report discomfort due to the slight stretching of the cervix that occurs as the IUD is passed into the uterus. Uterine cramps and dizziness are common, but generally subside quickly.

A woman should be examined following her first menstrual period after insertion, because the uterus is particularly likely to expel the device during this time. Many women learn to feel for the string protruding from the cervix to check the IUD's placement. Twice-yearly examinations are suggested as well. If a pregnancy should occur, the IUD must be removed immediately because of the possibility of serious pelvic infection. If the IUD is removed early and the pregnancy is desired, the pregnancy may be safely continued. However, the risk of miscarriage in these situations is higher than normal.

One of the complications associated with the use of intrauterine devices is the development of infection. Pelvic inflammatory disease (PID) may occur after the insertion of an IUD. The rate of PID in IUD users in general may be as much as five times normal. Multiple sex partners increase the infection risk as well—with or without an IUD. Infections may be very mild to quite severe, and can be caused by a number of different organisms. They can also be difficult to diagnose. For these reasons, as I have said, it is not my contraceptive of choice for women who desire a pregnancy in the future.

IUDs may also increase the incidence of ectopic pregnancies, that is, pregnancies that occur *outside* the uterus, most often in a Fallopian tube. There is no evidence at this time that any types of cancers are associated with the use of the IUD. It continues to be one of the most effective forms of birth control for the right woman at the right time.

LESS-EFFECTIVE APPROACHES TO BIRTH CONTROL

☐ *Rhythm,* despite its relative ineffectiveness, may be the only option available to some women because of their religious scruples. To complete the existing options, I am including an outline of the rhythm method of birth control. However, a woman who must not become pregnant, because of medical or emotional reasons, should not use this method. And a woman with irregular cycles cannot rely upon it.

This method is based on the fact that conception occurs at the time of ovulation, which is usually fourteen days before the onset of the next menstrual flow. A woman is, therefore, least likely to conceive at the beginning and the end of the menstrual cycle. A woman with a twenty-eight-day cycle should be able to have sex from days one to seven. The unsafe period is days eight to nineteen, followed by another safe time from day twenty to the onset of her period (Figure 8).

Some women add temperature-taking to simply counting the days of their cycles. A woman's morning temperature rises after ovulation,

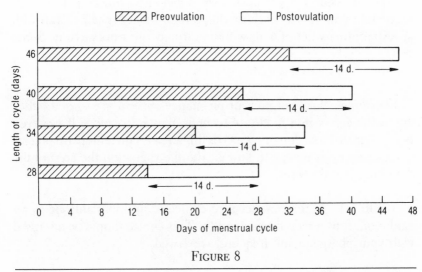

FIGURE 8

Ovulation occurs fourteen days before your period no matter what the length of the menstrual cycle.

due to the release of the hormone progesterone. If you take your temperature before getting out of bed each morning, using a special thermometer with fine gradations, then a fairly accurate determination of ovulation can be achieved. One can then assume that three days after the rise in temperature (usually to over 98° Fahrenheit) an egg released at ovulation will no longer be viable and the safe time has begun. There is also a method by which women track the monthly changes in cervical mucus, refraining from sex when the mucus signals fertility by becoming thin, slippery, and stretchy.

Unfortunately, ovulation times may vary. Even in fairly regular women, stress, weight changes, and numerous other physical and emotional occurrences can throw off the menstrual cycle. Another problem is that this system requires a long period of sexual abstinence during the so-called unsafe period. Your physician can guide you and teach you the method if you must use it.

☐ *Coitus interruptus:* Withdrawal of the penis before ejaculation is another ineffective method, though one of the oldest. This option is difficult to use and its failure rate is high. With this "method," sexual intercourse proceeds until just before the man reaches orgasm. As he feels orgasm coming, he pulls his penis from the vagina so no sperm are spilled inside the woman's body. Obviously, however, this technique relies on the use of sheer willpower. Why chance it? Even with an extraordinary act of will, withdrawal may not work anyway: Some sperm may be released *before* orgasm. It certainly doesn't lead to a fulfilling and relaxed sex life.

☐ *Douching* does not prevent pregnancy. Sperm are so quick they zip to the cervix in a matter of seconds after ejaculation. It has even been suggested that douching speeds this already efficient sperm process by pushing wayward sperm farther into the vagina on the crest of the douching liquid's wave.

In summary, your contraceptive choice is an important one as regards your future reproductive health. This choice should be discussed with your physician and frequently reviewed.

5

The Obstetrician/ Gynecologist: The Woman's Physician

The expert who cares for a woman's reproductive health through a lifetime of sexual partners, menstrual upsets, infections, birth control methods, pregnancies, and menopause treatments is called an "obstetrician/gynecologist." He or she is the woman's health care specialist: a physician with special training and surgical skills in women's health care. In addition to a medical school education and postgraduate training, the ob/gyn may have further credentials in the field. The specialist may be "board certified," meaning that he or she has successfully passed a special examination conducted by the American Board of Obstetrics and Gynecology. There are also "specialty boards" that signify additional training and accreditation in particular areas within obstetrics and gynecology, such as oncology (cancer) and endocrinology.

Gynecology encompasses all the areas of health care involving a woman's reproductive organs: choosing among birth control options, screening for and treatment of infection, cancer and other disorders of the female reproductive organs and breasts, treatment for infertility, premarital and sexual counseling, treatment of sexually transmitted disease, and therapy for conditions related to the menopause and postmenopausal years. Obstetrics is the care of a woman from the time she conceives through pregnancy, labor, delivery, and the healing phases after childbirth.

For many young women, their ob/gyn is also their "primary care physician"—a role that might otherwise be filled by a general practitioner, family doctor, or internist. The ob/gyn is often the only doctor with whom they have regular contact and a continuing relationship from the time they become sexually active until their middle years. As a primary physician the obstetrician/gynecologist evaluates a woman's overall health, cares for those problems within the specialty itself, and refers her, when indicated, to other physicians in other medical specialties.

Several sources of information can help you pick your obstetrician/gynecologist. These include your local medical society, your local hospital or medical school, your family physician, any other person whose judgment you trust, and the American College of Obstetricians and Gynecologists at 600 Maryland Avenue S. W., Suite 300 East in Washington, D.C. 20024.

ROUTINE GYNECOLOGIC CARE

A woman should start to have regular gynecologic examinations once she begins to have sex, or by the age of eighteen to twenty-one even if she's not sexually active. A female child or adolescent with a condition involving her reproductive system may need to see a gynecologist regardless of her age, and may be referred by a pediatrician. Besides routine gynecologic examinations, you should seek gynecologic care if you have significant changes or problems involving your reproductive organs. Obstetrical care should begin as soon as a woman first decides to have a baby—even *before* she becomes pregnant, so that she may plan in advance—sometimes years in advance—for an eventual healthy pregnancy and a healthy baby.

Being reproductively healthy is a responsibility shared by your physician and yourself. It is your responsibility to pay attention to your body and be alert to changes that suggest that something may be wrong. It is your doctor's responsibility to help you stay well and care for any problems that may occur. Keeping healthy involves cultivating good habits—eating nutritiously, getting adequate rest and exercise—and avoiding bad habits such as heavy drinking, smoking, and drug-taking, knowing your body and being receptive to its signals, and, of course, having regular checkups.

The gynecologic exam is the cornerstone of good reproductive health. Clearly, periodic examinations and testing can pick up changes early enough to treat them most effectively. The frequency of routine visits depends on the plan your doctor works out with you. Usually, he or she will want to see you at least once a year.

You should also see the ob/gyn between checkups when you experience major changes in your life. Some of the reasons for seeking care include vaginal discharge or irritation, contraceptive advice when you first become sexually active, and if there are problems with your method later, painful intercourse, menstrual cramps, and pregnancy planning.

THE OFFICE VISIT

A routine examination lets you be evaluated as a total person. It will consist of a family health history, personal health history, general physical examination, pelvic examination, education and counseling on reproductive health topics, and laboratory tests. The health history will include information about past illnesses, diseases, medical care, allergies, drug use, and hospitalizations, and may include a menstrual, sexual, contraceptive, and reproductive history. A family health history is important in terms of genetic problems that could be inherited, as well as problems that simply tend to run in families—high blood pressure, diabetes, heart disease. Remember, though, that every person is a unique individual: You will not necessarily follow the same health course as your relatives. It's good to know about the possibilities, nonetheless.

A physical examination usually begins with measurements of your weight and blood pressure. Blood pressure should be checked on a regular basis, since it can be elevated with no outward symptoms whatsoever. Caught early, high blood pressure can be treated before it has a chance to damage the heart, circulatory system, or kidneys. The doctor will generally check your heart and lungs, as well as your head and neck. Your breasts will be examined for signs of cysts or tumors. This examination should supplement your own monthly breast examination, so ask the doctor to show you how to do your own exam at home. (See, too, Chapter 2, "The Breast.")

Following the general external examination, an internal pelvic examination will be done. Although you may feel awkward lying on your back on the examination table with your feet up in the stirrups, this internal exam should not be painful. However, if you are very tense you may feel some discomfort. I try to get women to take a few deep breaths before I start, and I explain everything I do as I go along to help them relax as much as possible.

An instrument called a "speculum," shaped like a duck's bill and made of either plastic or metal, is used to hold the walls of the vagina apart so the vagina and cervix (the "neck" of the uterus, which protrudes into the top of the vagina) can be seen. While the speculum is in

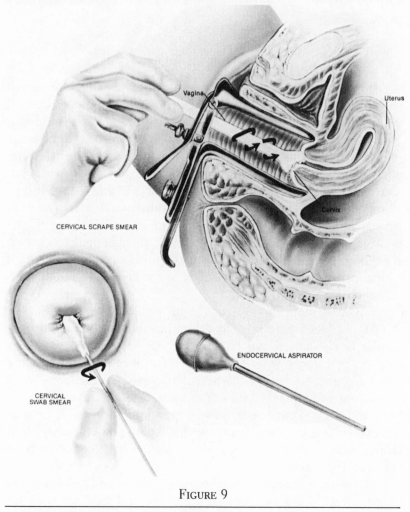

FIGURE 9

Technique for Papanicolaou ("Pap") test and speculum examination. Endocervical aspirator is sometimes used to obtain cells in the cervical canal. Courtesy of Syntex Laboratories, Inc.

place, a Pap smear will also be obtained (Figure 9). This involves gently scraping a few cells from the opening of the cervix and from the internal canal of the cervix with a small wooden or plastic spatula. These cells are then sent to a laboratory to be examined for evidence of infection or cancer. The Pap test is unique in that it can diagnose cancer at such an early stage that the cancer may be completely cured before it advances. A woman should have a Pap test every year, particularly if she started having sexual relations before age twenty, or has had several sex partners. (Cancer of the cervix is discussed in further detail in Chapter 8, "Gynecologic Problems.")

Next a "bimanual," or two-handed, pelvic examination is performed (see Figure 10). The doctor gently inserts two gloved fingers into the vagina and presses the other hand on the outside of the lower abdomen. The shape of the internal organs can be felt between the two hands, so that abnormalities of the uterus and ovaries, such as tumors or cysts, can be detected. The doctor may also then insert one finger in the rectum, leaving one in the vagina, for a more complete examination of the vagina itself, its surrounding structures, and the ovaries. Don't be disconcerted if this pressing and poking makes you feel the urge to urinate or move your bowels—the feeling stops as soon as the exam is complete, and is perfectly normal.

If the doctor has asked you for a urine sample, a urinalysis may be

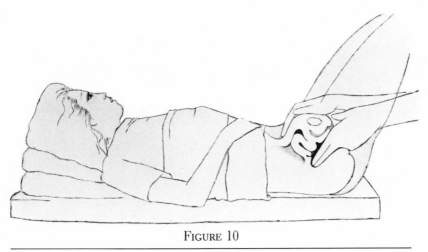

FIGURE 10

Bimanual internal pelvic examination

done to check for protein or sugar in the urine. Sugar may be evidence of diabetes; protein could indicate a kidney problem.

After taking the history, and doing the physical examination and the lab tests, the physician will usually ask you to get dressed and come to the office to discuss the results with you and answer any questions you may have. Feel free to bring up questions about birth control, pregnancy, genetic counseling, fertility, cancer signals, diet, exercise, and breast self-examination. Your doctor is there to answer your questions. Don't be embarrassed about "taking up time"; a few minutes of question-and-answer is a vital part of the exam for both you and your doctor.

Abnormalities such as infections, tumors, and cysts, if caught early, can often be treated effectively. This may avoid future problems both in conceiving and in pregnancy, and may prevent a minor problem from becoming something more serious. It is important for a woman to choose a doctor who doesn't patronize her, whom she can trust, and with whom she personally feels comfortable. You may have to visit a few before you find the right reproductive health practitioner for you.

PART II

Reproductive Health Problems

Introduction

It is important for women to have a basic understanding of the kinds of gynecologic problems that tend to crop up during their childbearing years. Familiarity with them will enable you to be alert to the body's early warning signs, and prevent potentially disabling problems from developing further.

Many of the things you will be reading about in the chapters ahead sound complicated, serious, and scary. But most are, in fact, quite minor, easily treated—completely curable. Other, serious conditions can be prevented from worsening, or treated to whatever extent possible at the stage at which they are diagnosed. Even very serious problems—those with a real potential for threatening your fertility—can best be dealt with when found and treated as soon as possible. Most often, even these problems still allow a good chance of pregnancy, especially if you and your doctor tackle them with that goal in mind.

6

Sexual Function
and Dysfunction

A normal, healthy sex life is part of good health—good emotional
health *and* good physical health, since sexual problems can cause
emotional distress which can lead to impaired fertility, which rebounds
as greater emotional stress. Emotional stress from any source can even
prevent ovulation. Moreover, a couple with a happy sexual relationship
will probably be able to create a more loving environment in which
to raise a family.

Doctors are faced with complaints about sexual problems more frequently today than they were in the past. Men and women worry about
lack of desire, inability to perform, or difficulty in achieving orgasm.
Talking about it is due to both the increased acceptability of acknowl-
edging that these problems exist and greater understanding about the
causes and treatment of sexual problems.

In order to put sexual dysfunction in perspective, it's important to
understand the normal sexual cycle. The cycles of both females and
males can be divided into four phases

1. The excitatory phase. This is characterized by an increase of blood
   flowing into the pelvic blood vessels. This rush of blood produces
   erection in a man and vaginal lubrication and genital swelling in
   a woman. In addition, the pelvic organs shift position slightly—
   the uterus is pulled up and the vagina increases in size.
2. The plateau phase. This occurs at peak enlargement and vascular

engorgement of the pelvis, after the pelvic organs have moved into ready position. Immediately before orgasm in the male there is a period called "ejaculatory inevitability"—when it is no longer possible for him to stop ejaculation voluntarily. There is no comparable period in women. The female cycle can grind to a halt from internal or external distractions at any point. A twinge of pain, an upsetting thought, a ringing phone can all do it.

3. The orgasmic phase. Male ejaculation and female orgasm are physiologically similar, although it is important to note that the emotional reactions to orgasm may vary from individual to individual, and may be affected in any one person by the time and situation. But the physiologic process remains the same. Orgasm muscle spasms occur in the outer third of the vagina and in the uterus. The degree of contraction parallels the intensity of the orgasm the woman experiences.

4. The resolution phase. After orgasm, there is a decrease in the amount of blood in the pelvic area, a gradual return to the unexcited state, and, in the male, a so-called refractory period, during which time a new excitement phase (erection) cannot occur. Although there is considerable normal variation, this period of time generally increases with age. It may last just a few seconds for a teenager, and as long as several days for a man who is over seventy.

Women have no refractory phase, which can allow multiple orgasms to occur in rapid succession. Multiple orgasms, however, do not occur in all women; some women who are multiorgasmic may not be so all the time. A number of women do not reach orgasm at all. Some can reach orgasm only by masturbation or oral sex, but not by intercourse. There is no reason to believe that this is an unhealthy situation. It appears to be simply one variation on functioning within the range of normal.

SEXUAL DYSFUNCTION IN WOMEN

There is often misunderstanding about the classification of dysfunction in the female. "Frigidity" is a catch-all term, used for anything from a failure to be sexually stimulated to an inability to reach orgasm. Well-known sexual researcher Helen Kaplan's classification scheme of sex problems is based on the sexual response cycle just described.

□ *Sexual unresponsiveness* comes closest to the term "frigid." This inhibition of sexual arousal is basically a squelching of all sexual feeling. Women with this problem suffer from an impairment of the early part of the sexual cycle so that they do not have sufficient pelvic blood flow, or vaginal lubrication or expansion. It may stem from negative attitudes about sexuality in general, other psychological problems, or difficulties with a particular partner. Rarely is the cause physical.

□ *Orgasmic dysfunction* occurs when a woman can respond sexually but then does not reach orgasm. This, too, rarely has a physical basis. It occurs most often in women with unrecognized fear and anxiety about losing control during orgasm or unrealistic expectations about sexual performance. If, for example, a woman fears she is inadequate, anxiety may appear at the moment of impending orgasm and involuntarily inhibit this reflex. Anger toward one's partner, or depression arising from any cause, may also decrease orgasmic potential. Repressed anger is a common cause of sexual dysfunction.

□ *Vaginismus* is an involuntary contraction of the outer third of the vagina that makes intercourse painful or impossible. It may be due to a previously traumatic sexual experience or to an anatomical abnormality called an "imperforate hymen." In the latter case, the hymen— a piece of tissue near the vaginal opening—is so thick it will not allow sexual intercourse without severe pain. A pelvic examination can diagnose this, and a simple surgical incision can open the too-tight hymen.

□ *Painful intercourse,* or dyspareunia, is the most common female sexual problem. A careful pelvic examination may reveal abnormalities of the vagina, cervix, or uterus. Sometimes conditions of the Fallopian tubes or ovaries can also make sex uncomfortable. Painful intercourse may also be due to insufficient lubrication. Spending a little more time on foreplay should be encouraged to sufficiently excite a woman and stimulate lubrication.

Causes of sexual problems can be divided into physical and psychological. The physical causes follow.

☐ *General health problems* can include diseases of the heart or kidneys, infections, or cancer. The sexual upset is related to decreased sexual drive due to general weakness, pain, or depression brought on by the illness.

☐ *Pelvic problems* such as diseases, growths, or anatomic abnormalities can interfere with sexual pleasure. The gynecologic disease known as "endometriosis," scar tissue due to pelvic infection, imperforate hymen, or vaginal or cervical infections are just a few of the possible causes.

☐ *Surgery* in a pregnancy delivery can occasionally cause sexual problems, as, for example, in a difficult delivery requiring surgical repair, where the inelastic scar tissue that forms can limit the tissue's ability to expand during sex. Other types of surgery to the pelvic region can change the position of organs, leave scar tissue, or otherwise leave the area unable to respond to sex normally.

☐ *Drugs and medications* can affect sexual response directly and indirectly, either by affecting the nervous system or by changing blood flow to various organs. Alcohol, barbiturates, and marijuana can all, in small amounts, increase responsiveness. But too much has the opposite effect and leaves you sexually groggy. Medications prescribed for anxiety or depression have a similar two-way effect. They may improve sexual behavior as they ease paralyzing anxiety or lift numbing depression, but they have been reported to decrease the sexual appetite as well.

The psychological aspects of sexual dysfunction have been studied extensively by the sex-therapist team Masters and Johnson. Their approach has been to correct sexual problems by behavior modification, without worrying about digging up the often remote psychological causes. The goal is simply to relieve the sexual dysfunction symptom rather than accomplish a total overhaul of an individual's personality or a couple's relationship. Sexual responsiveness is extremely subtle and complex. We enjoy sex most when we are relaxed, undistracted, and not consciously monitoring our performance.

Some of the psychological factors causing sexual dysfunction are linked to early sexual attitudes and experiences. Simple misinformation, fear, belief in "old wives' tales," and unrealistic expectations can be carried from childhood without ever being corrected. Negative family or societal attitudes may produce guilt, anxiety, or dislike of certain sexual practices. A traumatic experience such as rape or incest can obviously have a negative impact on a person's ability to enjoy sex. Homosexual experiences may produce anxiety about sexual identity or choice of partners. Family or work stress, misunderstandings between partners, infidelity, or boredom dampens many couples' sex lives, as can differences in life stages or divergent interests.

Sexual symptoms are sometimes just the tip of the iceberg, but may prompt someone to seek help. Some of the major psychological disorders that can produce sexual problems are low self-esteem, dependency, depression, an exaggerated need for control, and severe communication problems.

TREATMENT OF SEXUAL DYSFUNCTION

Among a number of approaches to treating sexual dysfunction, the work of Masters and Johnson in the last decade has produced some of the most impressive results.

They use several general principles in their approach to therapy. One is that the sexual problem, *whatever* it is, is the shared responsibility of the couple. It is not acceptable to place blame or to focus responsibility on one partner or the other.

Another principle is that sex is seen as a way of sharing enjoyment and relaxing. Partners are encouraged to be spontaneous and less rigid in what they think of as acceptable sexual behavior and the times and places to have sex.

There is also an emphasis on the enjoyment of sensuality without requiring orgasm each time. Communication is emphasized; the pressure to actually have sex is off. In fact, sex is actually not *allowed* for some period of time, to reduce anxiety about performance. The couple is encouraged to understand, accept, even delight in each other's values, preferences, differences. They are shown how to touch and how to explore the process of giving and receiving pleasure. Specific technical suggestions, directions, and techniques may be suggested as well.

The goal of therapy is to create an undemanding and relaxed environment for pleasurable sexual interaction to occur. Women who are sexually unresponsive often defend themselves against erotic feelings because of guilt or fear of rejection. They need support for sensual expression; so specific practices are emphasized that produce pleasure without demand. It is important that a woman experience her own sexual feelings rather than try to respond according to expectations or rules.

Eventually, sexual intercourse is resumed, generally after four to ten sessions. Enough confidence will often have been restored so that the couple can resume sex with the woman feeling secure. Even after all this, negative reactions to the experience are common and may take time to work out.

To attack orgasmic dysfunction, a woman is helped to give up her need for controlling her response—to just let it happen. This takes time and is complex. A woman may be taught to bring herself to orgasm through masturbation or with a vibrator, provided that she is ready to accept this practice. Fantasies are encouraged. If she worries that they are inappropriate, she needs to be reassured that they are not "sick," regardless of their content.

In one study of anorgasmic women about 90 percent of women could achieve orgasm by masturbation after five weeks of therapy. After eight months, they were able to transfer their new-found talent to sexual intercourse with a partner. But approximately 8 percent of women do not have orgasms by any means. Another significant percentage achieve orgasm through means other than intercourse. For the woman who has never had an orgasm, the objective is to achieve that first one. Often this dispels the nagging fear that she is incapable of orgasm and smooths the road to further progress.

Women need to be active participants in their own sex lives, not subject to the sexuality of their partners. If there is a problem, it is the couple's problem, not the woman's alone. Best of all, something can be done about it. Sex is a very basic yet extraordinarily complex human need. It should be a source not of anxiety and tension, but of pleasure, contentment, and joy.

RESOURCES FOR SEX THERAPY

Your physician is your best guide on where to seek help. Many medical centers have sex therapy clinics, as well. Do proceed with caution in your selection. Ask a potential therapist about his or her training, qualifications, and experience. There are many poorly trained individuals practicing as sex therapists because there is no legal control over who can use this title. However, states do restrict unqualified people from calling themselves psychologists or psychiatrists. One professional organization that helps provide standards for sex therapists is the American Association of Sex Educators, Counselors and Therapists (AASECT), 133 E. 35th St., New York, N.Y. 10016.

7

Common Infections

Almost every woman will get a vaginal infection or irritation sometime during her life. Most women will have several. Vaginal infections are not usually serious, but there is no question that they can be uncomfortable and annoying. The word "vaginitis" is a general term used to describe any type of inflammation or irritation of the tissue that lines the vagina. The most common symptoms of this irritation are burning or itching of the vagina or the labia, along with some kind of abnormal discharge. Vaginitis can be caused by many different things and is, in fact, a major reason women end up in their gynecologists' offices.

YEAST INFECTION: MONILIASIS

Monilia, or yeast, is one of the most common problems of a woman's childbearing years, especially during pregnancy. Birth control pills also predispose women to yeast infections. The link here is probably that both pregnancy and the Pill can make the vagina, quite literally, "sweeter" (with an increased sugar content), providing an environment in which the yeast fungus thrives.

If a smear of the vaginal secretions is scrutinized under the microscope, the small fiberlike organism called *Candida albicans* can be easily spotted. This fungus is actually present in small amounts in many normal, healthy vaginas. It lives there peacefully, causing no symptoms at all, until something sets off a growing spree. Multiplying rapidly, the yeast then upsets the normal balance of vaginal organisms, eventually irritating the walls of the vagina. Besides pregnancy and the use of birth control pills, diabetes, emotional stress, poor diet, excessive douching, even irritation from vigorous sex can all trigger monilia.

Antibiotics, oddly enough, are also a villain from the point of view of yeast infections. When you take an antibiotic to wipe out, say, the bacterial invaders causing a sore throat, the drug also destroys bacteria throughout the body, including the "healthy" ones that inhabit the vagina. This gives the yeast the opportunity to rapidly multiply and cause vaginitis. To head this off, many physicians prescribe an anti-yeast medication at the same time as an antibiotic.

Yeast can be transmitted by intercourse, although men rarely get a symptomatic infection from the organism. Occasionally the fungus also lives in the lower bowel; and careless wiping after a bowel movement may reinfect the vagina.

The symptoms characteristic of moniliasis vary from woman to woman but in general are:

• severe itching and irritation about the labia, or lips of the vagina, which may become red, swollen, and dry to the touch (scratching may make the irritation worse);
• a discharge that is thick and white (a bit like yogurt) or lumpy (like cottage cheese) with a nondescript or "baking bread" odor;
• burning of the vulva during urination from the acidic urine touching the irritated skin.

Women often notice that symptoms generally crop up or intensify around menstruation. Menstrual flow is alkaline, which, once again, alters the chemical environment in the vagina and allows this fungus to proliferate.

Many types of medication are available to treat yeast. Vaginal creams and suppositories include Mycostatin, Monistat, Candeptin, and Sporostacin. Ointments or creams containing soothing steroids and anti-yeast agents may also be used externally to reduce irritation and itching of the vulva. However, these must be used *with* vaginal treatment, or the source of the infection won't be cleared up. Sex during treatment for this infection may make irritation worse: Hold off until you've let the oversensitive vagina heal.

If you are taking birth control pills and get severe recurrent infections it may be necessary to switch to another contraceptive. Pregnant women with recurrent flareups may not really be completely cured until after giving birth. In the meantime, treatment can help keep the problem under control and minimize symptoms, with no danger to the fetus. Yeast infections can interfere with conception by causing painful intercourse and perhaps producing a hostile environment for sperm.

Trichomonas Vaginitis: "Trich"

The tiny one-celled organism called "trichomonas," seen under a microscope, has a pear-shaped body with a powerfully lashing tail. This unusual organism appears to have no function in life except to cause the annoying and very common vaginal infection known as "trich." Trichomonas may invade the vagina, the ducts alongside the urinary tract, called Skeen's ducts, and the urinary tract itself.

Most women get the disease by having sex with an infected man. Unfortunately, men may unknowingly carry the organism since they may not have any symptoms of infection. The organism can hide under the foreskin of uncircumcised men and may be excreted in the secretions from the male prostate gland. The infection can also be transmitted by contact with underwear, bath towels, and douche apparatus that have been exposed to the organism.

The symptoms of trich appear four days to a week after exposure. The vaginal symptoms include itching and burning, and a discharge that can be anything from clear to thick and yellowish. The most clear-cut symptom is a distinct, disagreeable odor. In general, however, the symptoms of trich are usually less irritating than those caused by yeast.

Your physician usually diagnoses trich right in the office with a so-called wet-mount slide of vaginal secretions, which reveals the organisms zipping about, whipping their tails. In a man, diagnosis can be made by checking the first morning urine for these organisms.

Sexual partners must be treated at the same time to avoid reinfecting each other. The drug metronidazole (Flagyl) is very effective in wiping out trichomoniasis. You may be given eight pills to take in 24 hours or three pills a day for a week. (Recurrent infections are treated for the longer period of time.) The drug may produce unpleasant side effects such as a "furry" tongue, an odd taste in the mouth, and some nausea and diarrhea. Alcohol intensifies these effects and should be scrupulously avoided until treatment is complete. This type of vaginitis may also interfere with conception by creating a hostile environment for sperm.

HEMOPHILUS VAGINITIS

During the past few years a mild form of vaginal infection called "hemophilus vaginitis" has been seen more and more often. Hemophilus was once lumped in a kind of throwaway category called "nonspecific vaginitis." With the development of more accurate diagnostic techniques, this bacterium can now be identified and a specific diagnosis made. As many as 40 percent of all vaginal infections are now thought to be due to hemophilus, as opposed to just 20 percent pinned on trichomonas. As with trich, sex is the way it's usually passed from person to person. Symptoms show up approximately five to ten days later.

The vaginal discharge is different from trich or yeast. Severe burning and itching are not common, and the discharge often resembles a thin flour-paste with minimal odor. Women often come to the office not quite sure if they actually have an infection. Here again, a wet smear is used to diagnose the ailment on the spot. Although the organism itself is invisible, under the microscope special characteristic cells are quite easy to pick out.

An oral antibiotic, such as ampicillin, for five to seven days, or a vaginal medication, such as a sulfa antibiotic, for about ten days, effectively wipes out this minor bug. Treatment of your partner is essential to keep you from reinfecting each other.

CHLAMYDIA

Recently, reproductive system infections caused by *Chlamydia trachomatis* have gained a great deal of attention and concern in the medical community. This unusual organism can survive only as a parasite within other cells, feeding off the host cell's metabolic processes.

Chlamydia causes a wide array of problems, including vaginitis and cervical infections (called "cervicitis"). It can also travel up into the uterus and out through the Fallopian tubes to the ovaries, causing a form of pelvic inflammatory disease (PID). The incidence of low-grade chlamydia infections of the vagina, cervix, and pelvic organs has increased dramatically in recent years. Some experts feel chlamydia is now the most common sexually transmitted disease. In a study in one clinic this infection was 50 percent more common than gonorrhea.

Since chlamydia is a major cause of pelvic infection it is of particular importance to women who have not finished childbearing and wish to preserve maximum fertility potential. The infertility rate following acute infection of the Fallopian tubes depends on how many and what types of infection a woman has had. But the figures are daunting: A single nongonococcal tubal infection (a category which includes chlamydia) produces a 15 percent infertility rate, compared with 6 percent after an infection with gonorrhea. Two infections leave 35 percent of women infertile; three, a staggering 75 percent. Chlamydia also may be responsible for repeated flareups of pelvic infection in the years after an acute gonorrhea infection—the gonorrhea infection seems to leave the body more vulnerable to chlamydia infections.

It has, then, become important for the gynecologist to culture for chlamydia more frequently, since a low-grade infection may produce few symptoms and still do damage. And women with any of the symptoms should be checked and cultured by their physician as soon as possible. The symptoms include a vaginal discharge, minor irritation of the vagina, minor abdominal pain, pain on sexual intercourse, low fever, and a vague general feeling of not being well.

Though serious, chlamydia is, fortunately, quite simple to treat. The antibiotic tetracycline is very successful in eradicating the organism. Ease of successful treatment is one more reason for women and their physicians to develop a high degree of awareness of this infection. Your fertility is precious; do all you can to preserve it.

HERPES

In contrast to chlamydia, almost everyone is well aware of herpes. Sometimes, however, the fear surrounding this infection is actually far out of proportion to the actual pain, suffering, and damage it causes. In only a few clearly defined situations is herpes really the villain it's sometimes made out to be. Unfortunately, one of the potentially dangerous times to have a herpes outbreak is at the end of pregnancy, since a baby can catch the infection from its mother during delivery.

Infection of the labia or vulva by the virus called "herpes simplex" has become vastly more prevalent in the last decade or so. Herpes virus was named after the Greek word meaning "to creep," for its seeming ability to crawl along nerve pathways. Given its spread in our population today, a better description might be "to gallop." One of the earliest descriptions of this infection was recorded in 1736 in France. However, it was not until 1946 that the virus causing the sores was isolated. By the 1960s the different virus types—I and II—had been identified.

Herpes type II virus is the one primarily responsible for genital infections. Type I virus most often affects the area around the mouth—its outbreaks are often dubbed "cold sores," or "fever blisters." Approximately 80 to 90 percent of women with genital herpes have the type II virus. The remaining 10 to 20 percent with genital infections have type I virus.

More people have this virus than know it: By checking the blood for antibodies specific to these viruses, it has become clear that a person can be infected without recalling any outbreak. A recent study in Texas found that approximately 10 percent of patients in a private gynecologic practice and 22 percent of patients in a gynecology clinic in a county hospital had evidence in their blood of a prior herpes type II infection. In another study of 1,000 pregnant women, 35 percent had evidence of a previous infection. However, in less than 1 percent could the virus be found on the cervix when the women had no symptoms.

The infection is usually caught by direct contact with a herpes sore. (Less common, although possible, is its spread without a visible sore.) The infection usually starts as a cluster of small ulcers (shallow open sores) or blisters that spread around the external vaginal area. Chief symptoms are sensitivity of the infected area—pain, burning, and itching, and burning when urine touches the raw skin. The virus can also cause sores on the buttocks, around the anus, on the lower abdomen and low back, as well as internally on the vaginal walls and cervix. A breakout may be accompanied by a low-grade fever, and the glands in the groin may swell. The primary, or first, outbreak may take three to six weeks to heal, though it usually leaves no scarring as long as the sores don't become infected. However, the area may still "shed" virus—i.e., be infectious—for about a week after that.

After that first outbreak heals over, the virus may retreat ("creep," like its name) along certain nerves under the skin and lie dormant, or inactive. Recurrences or flareups are most likely from this "latent" infection, rather than by reinfection of new virus. One out of two women have a recurrence, usually at the same place, within six months after the initial infection heals, although recurrent outbreaks are usually much less severe. Healing occurs more quickly, too, within a week to ten days; and within a week of healing the spot is usually not shedding virus anymore, so infecting someone else is unlikely. The swelling of the lymph glands in the groin is also less severe with recurrent infections.

Many women can tell when they are going to have a new outbreak. "The spot begins to tingle, itch, then burn," one reports, "right where the sores will soon show up." (From this point on there is a chance of passing the infection if you have sex.) Sometimes pain radiates up the back and down the legs. Recurrences may be provoked by stress, or may recur at certain times of the menstrual cycle, and for many reasons that are simply not known. Other triggers include colds, fevers, exposure to ultraviolet light (including sun), digestive tract disorders, trauma, sexual intercourse, and emotional upset from any cause.

☐ *Diagnosis* is easy nine out of ten times, since your doctor can recognize primary herpes on the basis of your symptoms and what he or she sees upon examining you. The infection can be confirmed by a viral culture, or by taking a scraping from these sores and staining it to highlight certain characteristic cells. But the blood studies for antibodies indicate only an earlier infection by the virus, since it takes six weeks for the body to produce the antibodies.

Treatment of herpes, which used to be limited to easing symptoms with warm baths with cornstarch or wet compresses of Burrough's Solution (available at your pharmacy), has recently seen an exciting advance. A new prescription drug called Acyclovir, available both in a dab-on ointment form and a pill form, is quite effective in cutting short the duration of the primary infection as well as recurrent infections. For best results, treatment should be instituted as soon as possible following the onset of signs and symptoms. Pills, taken daily, help prevent recurrent outbreaks, although continuous pill-taking is approved for only up to six months. Unfortunately, there is no evidence that after six months flareups will be permanently prevented, since these pills are not a cure.

Herpes infection can be a difficult problem for women who are plagued by frequent recurrences, though, over time, flareups become less and less frequent. Eventually, the body's defenses seem to put the disease on pretty much permanent hold. But it is recommended that women with herpes infections have Pap smears twice a year. There is an association between cervical cancer and this virus that, although not proven, makes it prudent for women to have this simple test in exchange for peace of mind.

☐ *Herpes and pregnancy* make a risky combination for the fetus and newborn, who are very susceptible to herpes virus and infection, and can have serious consequences. While in the uterus, the fetus is not at risk except in primary infections of the mother. During delivery, however, the infant may pick up the virus if it is present. To guard against this, herpes cultures are done weekly during the ninth month of pregnancy. If there is a positive culture or a herpes sore, delivery will be done by cesarean section. Some experts recommend vaginal delivery, even if there are visible sores, if the amniotic fluid sac has been ruptured more than six hours. The premise is that by that time the uterus already contains virus. However, some studies indicate that even then cesarean delivery is preferable.

Breastfeeding is allowed with a positive herpes culture, as long as care is taken so the newborn doesn't come in contact with active maternal sores. For women with inactive herpes at delivery, no special precautions are necessary for either mother or infant.

CONDYLOMA ACCUMINATA: GENITAL WARTS

Genital warts are caused by a virus called "papilloma virus." Women of childbearing age are most susceptible to this virus, which is spread by sexual contact. Generally, symptoms are minimal except for the presence of warty nodules or masses. However, treatment is necessary, or the virus will continue to spread. In addition, some types of condylomata virus have recently been implicated as a possible cause of cervical cancer and may affect reproduction in women afflicted.

The labia are the most common site of genital warts, although growths may arise around the rectum, pubic area, and vulva. The sexual partner should also be checked for warts and treated if any are found. Chemicals such as podophyllin may be called on to destroy the warts; or they may be frozen off with cryosurgery; or a laser may be used to vaporize them. Sometimes warts can be stubborn and must be treated again and again.

Some women with warts who deliver vaginally may pass this virus to their newborn. A few cases of warty growths (papillomas) of the larynx have been reported in infants of mothers with vaginal warts. However, this appears to be an unusual occurrence.

URINARY TRACT INFECTIONS

The urinary tract is made up of the kidneys (which produce urine), the ureters (which transport that urine), the bladder (which is basically a storage sac), and the urethra (which takes the urine from the bladder to the outside world). Infection can occur anywhere along this route, but bladder infections, called cystitis, are the most common.

Women are far more prone to bladder infections than men, since the female urethra is so much shorter than the male's, which runs to the tip of the penis. Besides this anatomic-design reason, cystitis can result from irritation to the urethra and bladder during prolonged sexual intercourse (so-called honeymoon cystitis). Diet, drinking habits, and careless wiping after bowel movements may also play a part in susceptibility.

The symptoms of cystitis include burning on urination, the urge to urinate constantly, blood in the urine, and lower abdominal and back pain. "Once you've felt it, you never forget!" exclaimed one young woman who has had several attacks. The diagnosis is confirmed by examining the urine for infection-fighting white blood cells and by culturing (or growing) bacteria from the urine. Because symptoms are so uncomfortable your physician will usually start treatment with antibiotics even before the results of the urine culture come back from the lab. A drug called Pyridium may also be used to ease severe symptoms, since it quickly numbs the tissues of the urinary tract. It is important to continue taking the antibiotics for a full week even though symptoms may subside after a day or two. If you don't, the infection can bounce back, full force, from the bacteria the antibiotics didn't have a chance to kill.

Women who have cystitis or recurrent symptoms may be helped by the following:

- Drink lots of water, because it helps to flush bacteria out of the bladder and increase the concentration of the antibiotics in the urinary tract.
- Warm baths can be a great help in soothing irritated tissues.
- Alcohol, citrus fruits, coffee, caffeine-containing sodas, and sex all tend to irritate the bladder and make symptoms worse. As long as you're still uncomfortable, try to avoid them.
- Women who get cystitis frequently may be able to reduce recurrences

by urinating as soon as possible after sex. This may wash out bacteria that might have been pushed into the urethra.

- Wiping from front to back after a bowel movement helps keep bacteria in the stool away from the urethral opening.
- Women who use a diaphragm and get recurrent cystitis may be helped by changing to a smaller size. (A too-large diaphragm can squash the urethra and irritate it.) If that fails, it may be necessary to switch to another method of birth control.

Recurrent cystitis may require the use of antibiotics for a long time (as long as six months) to keep the urine sterile and kill off the last vestiges of bacteria hiding out within the inflamed urinary tract tissues. Although common, cystitis should not be taken lightly; appropriate treatment should always be given to prevent chronic infections. Before becoming pregnant, women who have had recurrent urinary tract infections should have a urine culture done, even if they have no symptoms at the time. Recurrence of infections is more likely during pregnancy, which can affect the fetus. Women with chronic urinary tract infections tend to have smaller babies; prematurity and kidney infections are more common. Therefore, it is important that the urinary system be thoroughly checked by your physician both before and during pregnancy.

BARTHOLIN'S DUCT INFECTIONS

The two small glands, one on each side of the vaginal opening, called "Bartholin's glands," secrete mucus that is partially responsible for the lubrication that occurs during sexual arousal. When some type of infection blocks one of the ducts leading from these glands, a Bartholin's cyst may form. Gonorrhea is one infection that can plug up a Bartholin duct (usually only one gland becomes involved). With the duct blocked off, the gland itself gets swollen and may become infected—forming a large, painful, pus-filled lump. The cyst has then become a Bartholin abscess. An extremely large infected cyst can make walking, sitting, and sex uncomfortable. If the cyst stays small, a woman may have no symptoms. Or she may feel, at most, minor discomfort during sex. Diagnosis is made by examination of the labia, where the lump, large or small, can be easily felt.

The treatment of Bartholin cysts varies. A small, asymptomatic cyst can just be left alone. A painful abscess of the Bartholin gland may require an incision so it can drain. If there are recurrent abscesses, a simple surgical procedure called "marsupialization" may be performed. This technique, which can be done in the doctor's office after the acute infection is cleared up, preserves the function of the gland while preventing the formation of any new cysts or abscesses.

PUBIC LICE: "CRABS"

A tiny (1.5-millimeter), dark gray bug called the crab louse, or, more correctly, *Phtirius pubis*, may take up residence in human pubic hair and dine on human blood. Crabs come under the heading of sexually transmitted diseases since they most often hop from an infected person to his or her partner during sex. They are sometimes acquired from bedding or toilet seats as well. Severe itching heralds their arrival, and scratching can be severe enough to cause sores in this area. Diagnosis is confirmed by examining the base of the hairs for eggs (or nits) that female lice cement to the shafts. Grown crabs may be spotted hiding among the hairs, but tend to dash away before you're sure you've even seen them.

Highly effective shampoos are available over the counter to kill lice. It is important that all sexual partners be treated as well to prevent reinfection, and that all underwear, sheets, nightgowns, or other garments coming in contact with the pubic area be thoroughly washed in hot water and detergent. This infection does not affect pregnancy or fertility.

VENEREAL DISEASE

A venereal disease is simply an infection that is passed along most often from sex with an infected person. (The word "venereal" is derived from Venus, the Roman goddess of love.) Until recently, VD tended to refer mostly to gonorrhea or syphilis. But over the past few years, an increasing number of infections affecting the vagina, cervix, and penis have been recognized as being transmitted primarily by sex. As we have already seen in this section, herpes, trichomonas, condylomata, hemophilus vaginitis, and chlamydia are all known to be passed by sexual contact.

In the past, the term "venereal disease" carried certain implications; VD was, somehow, more than a disease. Leftover assumptions of the social status and respectability of those who got venereal diseases persist even today. Slowly, however, greater education in this area and preventive measures are starting to change its image. Also, partially to avoid the stigma of VD, the phrase "sexually transmitted disease" is being substituted. People find this phrase less frightening and less laden with the connotations of immoral living, which kept people from getting adequate treatment and cure. Gonorrhea and syphilis can lead to serious illness, or sterility. Ironically, almost all of these ailments can be quickly and effectively cured—*if* they are caught in time. However, venereal diseases are not infections you can catch only once. More like the common cold, a sexually transmitted infection can be caught every time you're exposed to it.

Prevention and early treatment are the keys to minimizing the dangers of sexually transmitted diseases. The use of condoms, contraceptive foams and jellies, as well as the diaphragm all somewhat reduce the chances of infection. Avoiding sex with men who have specific symptoms—a discharge from or sores on the penis—as well as routine checkups with your physician are also important. Education and the prevention of sexually transmitted diseases are critical to preserving your future childbearing capabilities. Gonorrhea, when associated with pelvic inflammatory disease, can produce severe scarring of the Fallopian tubes and leave a woman infertile. Chlamydia, as I discussed earlier, also is associated with chronic pelvic inflammatory disease and a high risk of sterility. Avoidance of infection when possible, and early and adequate therapy when these problems arise, will give you the best chance of preserving your fertility.

GONORRHEA

Gonorrhea is one of the most common bacterial infections in the civilized world. Caused by a bacterium, *Neisseria gonococcus,* it is a disease that works its way gradually along the passages of the urinary and genital tracts. It is the oldest known sexually transmitted disease; early cases were described in Mesopotamia in 5000 B.C. Today it is estimated that 2 million cases of gonorrhea occur in the United States every year.

The epidemic spread of gonorrhea has been of enormous concern to public health scientists; the number of cases has risen steadily since 1958 and nearly doubled since 1965. Up to 10 percent of women in some family planning clinics are found to be infected. Over half these cases are women under twenty-one, their fertility in jeopardy before they are old enough even to think of having a family.

Worst of all, most women with gonorrhea have no noticeable signs or symptoms, but this so-called carrier can infect anyone she has sex with (including oral or anal sex). Men, on the other hand, are more likely to have symptoms that force them to seek treatment. Many women become aware of their infection only when the men they have slept with inform them that they have contracted the disease.

If there is an early symptom in women, it's likely to be a minor, puslike discharge from an infected cervix. Symptoms of cystitis may also occur—frequent, burning urination. As the infection spreads, the symptoms of pelvic inflammatory disease may arise—low fever, vague pelvic pain, tiredness. Besides the genital tract, gonorrhea may also invade the Bartholin glands, urinary tract, anus, and rectum.

Gonorrhea is diagnosed by your physician from the physical symptoms and appropriate cultures. It should be treated aggressively with antibiotics, in order to prevent damage to the Fallopian tubes. If the Fallopian tubes are damaged the passage of the eggs through them may be blocked or hampered, resulting in total sterility or a dangerous tubal pregnancy.

The treatment of choice for gonorrhea is high doses of penicillin. Other antibiotics, such as tetracycline, can be used for those allergic to penicillin. Adding a drug called Probenecid to the antibiotic treatment slows the speed at which your body excretes penicillin, so a high level stays in the blood for a longer period of time. It is important that cultures be repeated following treatment, to make sure the gonorrhea is wiped out. All sexual partners must be treated.

A pregnant woman with untreated gonorrhea may infect the baby during delivery. All fifty states now require that the eyes of newborns be treated with either an antibiotic or silver nitrate to prevent the blindness gonorrhea can cause. Pregnant women with gonorrhea can safely be treated with penicillin. They should not, however, receive tetracycline; erythromycin or a cephalosporin can be used for those allergic to penicillin.

Anyone known to have been exposed to gonorrhea should, in my opinion, be treated with a full dose of antibiotics. I recommend this even if, for some reason, the cultures come back negative. The risks of infection are too high, and the treatment is too simple, to take a chance on an incorrect test result.

SYPHILIS

Syphilis is caused by an organism called *Treponema pallidum*. It is spread through vaginal intercourse and oral and anal sex. The time from exposure to symptoms ranges from as few as nine to as many as ninety days. Unlike gonorrhea, syphilis does not occur in epidemic numbers; but, left untreated, it can be much more devastating.

Its effects on pregnancy can also be devastating. Syphilis can cause abortion, prematurity, stillbirth, and many congenital abnormalities. Every woman should be checked for syphilis early in pregnancy through the blood test described below.

The effects of syphilis are divided into stages. Primary syphilis is caused by the bacterium's actually being present in your body. A painless sore, called a "chancre," develops, which may pass unnoticed if it is hidden inside the vagina. The chancre of syphilis is harder to overlook in men because, on the penis, it is much more visible.

In three to eight weeks, after the organism has spread through the body, syphilis enters its second stage. Rashes may appear on the skin, and there may be headaches, fever, and a general unwell feeling. After this stage, the disease goes underground. Latent syphilis may remain asymptomatic, the organisms staying inactive for many years. Eventually, however, these organisms "reawaken," to produce devastating effects on various organs—the heart, brain, muscles, and more—and even cause death.

The diagnosis of syphilis is made most often by a blood test, since over half the time the initial chancre is not observed. During the primary stage, a so-called dark field examination of the chancre itself can reveal signs of the organism causing the disease. Six or so weeks after the primary chancre, antibodies can be identified in the blood as well.

A German scientist, August P. von Wassermann, was the man who developed the first blood test for syphilis. Even today this test is often termed a "Wassermann" test, although it has been modified in various ways over the years. Today a variation called the "VDRL" test (since it was developed by the Venereal Disease Research Laboratory) is the one most commonly used. In many states, it *must* be performed before a marriage license can be obtained. The VDRL test shows positive no matter what stage the syphilis is in. However, it is not very "specific"—meaning other disorders such as mononucleosis, chicken pox, and lupus can give a false-positive VDRL result. When this happens, other more specific tests can be used to confirm or overturn the diagnosis of syphilis.

As with gonorrhea, it is vitally important that all sexual contacts be notified and treated even if no evidence of the disease can be found. Syphilis can be cured in any stage, although the damage caused by the third stage is irreversible. It is one of the few very serious infections with such a high cure rate. However, early diagnosis is important to avoid transmitting the disease to others and to make sure it is caught before pregnancy. Penicillin is the drug of choice to treat syphilis; it is very effective. Again, for those allergic to penicillin, tetracycline is an alternative. Follow-up blood tests should be performed to make sure that the infection is cured.

LESS COMMON VENEREAL DISEASES

Besides the common sexually transmitted diseases I've described, there are three others that are much less widespread, but that should be mentioned. They don't directly affect reproduction but have general health implications.

Lymphogranuloma venereum (LGV) is caused by the chlamydia organism and is spread by sex. In this case, the chlamydia get into the lymphatic system—the network of fluid filters found throughout the body—and causes a hard, painful lump in the groin. This swelling can break through the skin and drain. Diagnosis can be made by a special skin test called a "Frei" test. The antibiotic treatment is tetracycline for approximately one month. LGV occurs most frequently in homosexual men; if the infection is not treated, scarring of the anus can occur. Fewer than 500 cases are reported in the United States each year.

A second minor venereal disease is called "chancroid." Chancroid is caused by a small bacterium that infects the skin around the vulva or penis. At first, small blisters appear and break down into tiny ulcers; then the nearby lymph glands can become inflamed. Although it is difficult to distinguish this disease from herpes by examination, diagnosis can be made by culture from the sores. Sulfa antibiotics or tetracycline can cure it.

A third minor sexually transmitted disease is called "granuloma inguinale." It is caused by a bacterium that is common in southern climates and is characterized by blisters or sores in the genital area. Its diagnosis is made microscopically by spotting a particular structure called a "Donovan body" in the infected tissue. Tetracycline or ampicillin clear up this relatively uncommon infection.

AIDS

Acquired immune deficiency syndrome (AIDS) is the advanced stage of an infection which is caused by a virus, HTLV-III. This virus mainly attacks the T-cells—specialized blood cells that normally mobilize the immune system when a foreign invader strikes. However, once this virus enters these cells it commandeers them for its own use—turning them from defenders against disease into virus factories. Once all the T-cells are destroyed by the virus the immune system of the body is greatly weakened, and the body is open to all kinds of infections that previously would have been fought off with ease. It is these so-called opportunistic infections (including Kaposi's sarcoma, pneumocystis pneumonia, and other rare infections), not AIDS itself, that eventually kills AIDS victims.

The AIDS virus is passed from person to person by sex or by blood contamination. The vast majority of AIDS patients in the United States so far have been gay or bisexual men. However, the number of "straight" men or women getting the disease seems to be rising. Most of these latter have been users of intravenous drugs, or have received blood transfusions contaminated with the virus, or were sexual partners of infected individuals, or children born to infected mothers.

Recently, the AIDS virus has been isolated from vaginal and cervical secretions, confirming what many have suspected—that female genital secretions may be one source of transmission of the virus to men. Two separate studies, one in Boston and one in San Francisco, have succeeded in culturing (growing) the virus from the genital secretions of women at risk for the disease, meaning that they either were prostitutes, had partners with the disease, or had a history of intravenous drug use. Until now, male-to-male sexual transmission has been the principal means of infection in the United States and Europe, although in Africa and Haiti the disease is spread heterosexually. While the amount of virus found in the vaginal secretions of the women studied was low, it does suggest that the transmission of the disease from women to men through normal vaginal intercourse is possible, if uncommon.

The incubation period—how long it takes the disease to show up after you get it—is not known. Men who have had homosexual sex in the past eight years are advised not to give blood, since the virus may be dormant for a long period. Women seem to have caught the disease from a male partner who also had homosexual encounters or who was "shooting up" (injecting drugs). Such a man may not necessarily have symptoms, but can still have the deadly virus circulating in his blood.

AIDS-Related Complex (ARC) is a less serious form of the disease, in which swollen glands, weight loss, fatigue, and a persistent sore throat occur. Not all people with ARC develop full-blown AIDS. People with ARC are infectious, but this disease is not fatal if AIDS does not develop. There are also many people with HTLV-III virus in their bloodstream who have no symptoms of AIDS or ARC at all.

A blood test that checks for the presence of antibodies against the HTLV-III virus is very sensitive (98 percent effective in finding the antibodies) but it is not very specific. False positives frequently occur, especially in women who have had several pregnancies or who are on birth control pills. A more complicated and more specific test is available, which, although impractical to use as a general screen, can be performed if there is a positive antibody result.

At this time there is no known way to vaccinate against AIDS or to treat it effectively. Its spread may be curtailed as people become educated about the way it is transmitted—almost exclusively through sex (especially anal sex) and the use of shared needles by drug users. Anal intercourse, oral sex during which semen is swallowed, and any other practice that involves an exchange of body fluids can be dangerous.

If you do have casual sex, ask prospective partners about homosexual experiences or intravenous drug use. If they've had either in the past eight to nine years, they may have been exposed to AIDS. Condoms may be somewhat protective, but common sense is really your best weapon against this disease. All studies emphasize the need for safe sexual practices through avoiding high-risk partners and not being promiscuous.

8

Gynecologic Problems

Conception and pregnancy are complex processes that can be affected by various types of gynecologic problems. This chapter will outline some of the more common types of complaints of women in their childbearing years. Some of these problems have a more direct effect on reproduction than others. But no matter how tenuous the connection may seem at times, the fact remains that good gynecologic health is intrinsic to preserving your fertility and maintaining your ability to bear a healthy baby.

ENDOMETRIOSIS: THE CAREER WOMAN'S DISEASE

Endometriosis is a disorder of the female reproductive system that occurs only during the years of menstruation. Many women who have endometriosis have absolutely no symptoms. However, undetected and untreated endometriosis can cause severe damage to reproductive organs, resulting in infertility. For the many women who have postponed pregnancy, this disorder is a negative factor in their continuing reproductive potential. It is sometimes called "the career woman's disease" since it is most common in women in their thirties and forties who have not had children and who work in high-stress jobs.

Endometriosis occurs when tissue that essentially looks and acts like endometrium (the lining of the uterus) grows outside the uterine cavity. It is thought to occur when endometrial tissue that is shed during menstruation somehow flows backward—through the Fallopian tubes and out into the abdominal cavity. This tissue can then, apparently, implant and grow—on the *outside* of the uterus, in the tubes and on the ovaries, or on other nearby organs like the bladder and bowel (see Figure 11).

Each month the misplaced endometrial tissue responds to the changing hormonal patterns of the menstrual cycle, just like the normal uterine lining; and at the end of each cycle the endometriosis will shed and bleed. The blood and tissue, with nowhere to go, will cause irritation and local inflammation, and eventually leave scars behind. Month after month, patches of endometriosis "menstruate" and add to the damage. Sometimes the endometriosis eventually burns itself out without extensive damage. In other cases it continues to bleed and spread, causing new areas of disease and scarring.

How does endometriosis produce infertility? Besides scarring and

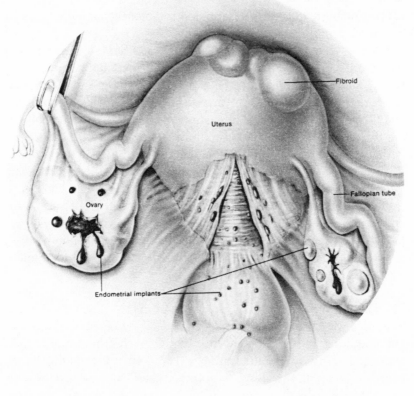

FIGURE 11

Common sites of endometriosis include the uterus, rectum, and Fallopian tubes. Courtesy of Syntex Laboratories, Inc.

disfiguring the Fallopian tubes and ovaries, the secretions from the misplaced tissue itself may possibly affect the process of fertilization. However, treatment of infertility due to endometriosis often has excellent results.

☐ *The signs and symptoms of endometriosis* include the common early symptom of increasingly painful periods, called dysmenorrhea. Painful intercourse, or dyspareunia, may result from endometriosis that has grown in the space behind the cervix at the top of the vagina. This area may be scarred and become tender and swollen around the time of the menstrual cycle, resulting in deep pain on sexual intercourse. Discomfort may occur in the bladder or in the lower intestines or bowel; and urinary frequency or painful bowel movements may be more pronounced around the time of the menstrual cycle. Unexplained inability to conceive is another symptom—often the first sign that something is amiss.

No one knows what triggers endometriosis. Some experts suspect that the delay of pregnancy into the thirties may be a contributing factor. Heredity is thought to be another factor. On the other hand, pregnancy and breastfeeding, because they stop menstruation for months, often have a beneficial effect on endometriosis; pregnancy and delivery are thought to help prevent any future development of the disorder. Perhaps the stretching of the cervix that occurs during delivery makes it easier for menstrual flow to exit from the body, thereby reducing the risk of backflow. Birth control pills curtail development and spread of endometriosis—perhaps by their chemical mimicking of pregnancy, and the lining of the uterus is much thinner, too, in women who are taking birth control pills, so there is less to shed each month. Birth control pills are, in fact, sometimes used to control and treat endometriosis.

☐ *Diagnosing endometriosis* may be as simple as a pelvic examination. If a woman comes to her doctor with any of the symptoms of endometriosis, the gynecologist may be able to confirm the early signs at once. There may be a thickening and tenderness behind the uterus, or irregularities and swelling around the tubes and ovaries. However, in most cases a final, accurate diagnosis is established only by a procedure called a "laparoscopy." This involves inserting a small telescopelike instrument through a small incision in the navel, and scrutinizing pelvic organs for any endometriosis scars or growths. (For more on this see Chapter 23, "Infertility Tests.")

☐ *The treatment of endometriosis* has an excellent success rate. Several methods of hormonal treatment have been developed to combat it, falling into two general categories. One type of therapy mimics the hormones of pregnancy, causing periods to stop, which results in the eventual shrinking of the endometrial patches. Birth control pills are used on a continuous basis (i.e., taken without the usual "off" week) in this type of hormonal therapy. The other type of therapy, using a drug called Danocrine, shuts down the menstrual cycle by simulating a temporary menopause. Many successful pregnancies have resulted from these approaches.

Surgery is also used to treat endometriosis. Large growths around the tubes and ovaries can be cut away with a scalpel. Cysts as big as grapefruits have been removed this way! Lasers and electrocautery can vaporize or burn away small spots of endometriosis. Surgery is followed by hormonal therapy to keep the disease from recurring. Surgical treatment of endometriosis has not been as popular since the development of effective hormone regimens. The decision to have surgery is an individual one and is best decided with your gynecologist.

The *best* treatment for endometriosis is prevention in the form of regular checkups. Your gynecologist may pick up the early signs of endometriosis and get therapy going *early*, so extreme spread of the disorder can be arrested and fertility preserved.

ABNORMAL UTERINE BLEEDING

Most women will have some abnormality in their periods during their childbearing years: bleeding too frequently, too long, or between cycles. Some of these symptoms may signal problems that could affect your ability to conceive. What constitutes abnormal bleeding?

For starters, it is very difficult for you or your physician to estimate the amount of your menstrual flow. Also, an amount that is perfectly normal for one woman may be totally out of line for another. Therefore, one of the best ways to determine if menstrual flow is too profuse for *you* is to have a blood count to see if the blood loss is producing anemia. As long as your health is unimpaired there is usually little reason to be concerned about minor menstrual changes. However, frequent bleeding between menstrual cycles, very irregular, profuse bleeding, or profuse regular periods should be checked out.

The most common reasons for abnormal bleeding are usually what experts call "functional," meaning they are not associated with a physical disease. It is important, however, that functional bleeding be a "diagnosis of exclusion"—in other words, physical diseases must be ruled out first. Growths like fibroids or polyps of the uterus (which will be discussed later) can cause an overly profuse menstrual flow. During pregnancy abnormal bleeding can be caused by a threatened miscarriage or an ectopic pregnancy. In addition, various illnesses that affect the general body functions can produce abnormal menstrual function. In twenty- to thirty-year-olds, cancer is not a likely cause of uterine bleeding, but around menopause this becomes more of a concern.

An operation called dilatation and curettage (D&C) is the principal tool the gynecologist uses to both diagnose and treat abnormal bleeding. With this technique, the cervix is opened slightly and the uterus is gently scraped with a tool known as a "curette." From a D&C, the gynecologist obtains tissue from inside the uterus for examination under a microscope, and also feels the inside of the uterus for irregularities. Many physicians are now doing D&Cs on an outpatient basis (you'll be in and out of the hospital or your doctor's office the same day) using only local anaesthesia.

If a physical disease can be ruled out, then hormone therapy may be started to try to correct functional abnormal bleeding. It is important to remember, however, that this treatment should not be given until serious abnormalities, including cancer, have been ruled out. If you are uncertain whether or not vaginal bleeding is abnormal, consult your physician.

FIBROIDS OF THE UTERUS

One of the most common gynecologic ailments to appear during the later menstrual years are the benign, fibrous growths called "uterine fibroids." Fibroids can affect your reproductive potential; they can be associated sometimes with infertility, repeated miscarriages, or difficulty with vaginal delivery. Approximately one in five women over the age of thirty will have some fibroids. Although they are more common in the late thirties and the forties, some women do get them as early as their twenties. These growths vary widely in size, shape, and position in the uterus. Their growth is sparked by hormones, particularly estrogen, and progesterone to a lesser extent. Fibroids usually shrink after menopause because of lack of stimulation from these ovarian hormones, which were formerly manufactured by the body.

There are three basic types of fibroids, categorized by where they grow in the uterus (see Figure 12). Fibroids within the muscular walls of the uterus are called "intramural." This most common type of fibroid can grow quite large. Generally asymptomatic when small, once they swell to the size of a three- to four-month pregnancy they can press on the bladder or the rectum and cause lower abdominal discomfort.

The second, less common type of fibroid, called "subserous," grows on the outside surface of the uterus. They, too, can become quite large, but are less likely to produce symptoms than the intramural type.

The third type of fibroid, located in the lining of the uterus, or endometrium, is called a "submucus" fibroid. These are the least common type, but produce symptoms even when very small. Because of their location in the endometrium, they can interfere with menstrual

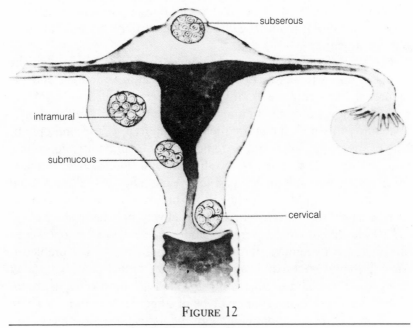

FIGURE 12

Basic types of uterine fibroids.

function and cause excessive bleeding. If weakness and anemia occur, these fibroids will require treatment. In addition, submucus fibroids may interfere with fertilization or implantation, causing infertility or miscarriages.

The work-up for infertility and repeated miscarriages will include diagnostic tests to rule out the presence of these abnormal growths. Larger fibroids can often be felt during a pelvic examination; but small submucus fibroids cannot be diagnosed this way, and may require a D&C. Another diagnostic technique is called "hysteroscopy." This involves inserting a tiny periscopelike instrument through the cervix and into the uterus to look for any irregularities in the endometrium. A third way to diagnose fibroids is with an x-ray technique called a "hysterogram"; injecting x-ray-visible dye into the uterine cavity will show up irregularities on the endometrium surface on the film. (This technique will also reveal if the Fallopian tubes are open, as will be explained in Chapter 23, "Infertility Tests.")

The treatment of fibroids depends on the symptoms. Their presence alone does not indicate a need for surgery. The basic concept that fibroids regress after menopause is important in determining appropriate treatment. Subserous and intramural fibroids rarely require surgery unless they become very large or produce pressure symptoms. Submucus fibroids producing bleeding, miscarriage, or infertility may require surgery.

The type of surgery needs to be individualized, depending on the woman's age, whether or not a future pregnancy is desired, and the nature of the symptoms. Conservative surgery, called a "myomectomy," removes only the fibroids and leaves the uterus intact. A hysterectomy, in which the entire uterus is removed, is a second option. The ovaries may or may not be removed at the same time, depending upon other factors. The conservative myomectomies have become more widely available in the past few years. They will allow normal pregnancy and childbirth; although if fibroids were extensive and the uterine cavity was entered, a cesarean delivery may be necessary.

I would like to offer a word of caution here: Too often operations are suggested to remove fibroids that are not causing any problems. Most fibroids do not require surgery. Remember that they regress after menopause, are almost always benign, and are most often asymptomatic. A second opinion for *any* type of surgery is appropriate. There are often differences of opinion about the indications for surgery even between good, well-meaning gynecologists. Many medical insurance companies recognize this and will often pay for the second opinion. Some even *require* them for hysterectomies.

OVARIAN GROWTHS

An understanding of various types of ovarian growths is important because many women encounter this diagnosis during their child-bearing years, and some forms can directly affect the ability to conceive. The ovary is one of the most active organs in the body. During the first half of the menstrual cycle, for example, several small, fluid-filled cysts form, each containing an egg. Usually one egg is released and the other cysts simply disappear. Sometimes, however, these cysts do not regress, but grow. They may cause pain and throw off the regularity of the menstrual cycle.

Ovarian cysts can often be felt by your gynecologist in a pelvic examination (see Figure 13). While most benign cysts will disappear with time, your gynecologist is faced with the problem of differentiating them from more serious types of ovarian enlargements, both benign and malignant. Therefore, if a cyst of 5 cm or greater is discovered, further testing—a sonogram or an x-ray, for example—may be ordered. Occasionally laparoscopy can be of value in making a diagnosis. If there is a strong possibility the cyst is benign, the gynecologist may suppress menstruation with hormones over a couple of months, to see

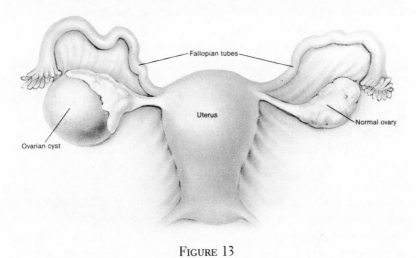

FIGURE 13

An ovarian cyst
Courtesy of Syntex Laboratories, Inc.

if the lump will get smaller. Unfortunately, surgery sometimes is required to make a definitive diagnosis. Benign cysts cannot always be differentiated from malignant cysts on the basis of physical findings or tests alone. The only really definitive diagnosis comes from examining the tissue of the lump itself, in a lab, under a microscope. Most benign ovarian cysts will not affect pregnancy potential. However, endometriosis can present itself as an ovarian growth. Malignant growths require removal of the ovary.

PELVIC PAIN

One of the most common, and most difficult, problems seen by gynecologists is lower abdominal pain. Most women will attribute pain in the lower abdomen to their reproductive organs. At least 60 percent of the time they are wrong. Some causes of abdominal pain can affect your fertility, however. Pelvic inflammatory disease and endometriosis are two causes that create touchy problems in reproduction.

Diagnosis of pain in the lower abdomen is complicated by the number of organs packed into this area. Besides the reproductive organs, there is the urinary system, the colon, and even part of the small intestine. The list of what can go wrong to cause lower abdominal pain is, then, almost mind-boggling. Since most causes of pelvic pain are minor, it is important for women not to jump to the conclusion that they have a serious problem such as malignancy. Some of the pain-causing problems of the intestinal tract, for example, include constipation, appendicitis, inflammation of the large or small bowel (irritable bowel syndrome), and diverticulitis. In the urinary tract pain can be caused by infections, stones in the bladder or kidney, and difficulty in urination. Even muscle and bone pain—a ruptured disc in the lower back, poor posture, scoliosis, arthritis, or muscle inflammation—can be perceived as pelvic pain.

The varied causes of gynecologic pelvic pain are summarized below.

☐ *Ovarian cysts* generally are not painful. However, if they twist on their blood supply or become inflamed, severe pain, which may radiate into the thighs, may require immediate medical attention. Surgery may be necessary. Most ovarian cysts are benign, but any ovarian lump larger than 5 cm, even if not painful, must be evaluated by your physician.

☐ *Pelvic inflammatory disease* can cause severe pelvic pain, which may be either one-sided or diffuse in the lower abdomen. The severe pain commonly occurs after menstruation and is often associated with a vaginal discharge and fever. Pelvic inflammatory disease can also cause mild, chronic discomfort. The severe pain is usually due to recent exposure to organisms such as gonorrhea; the chronic pain may be due to intermittent flareups of an old infection from organisms like chlamydia (see Figure 14).

☐ *Mittelschmerz, or ovulation pain* can occur at ovulation, when a small amount of blood may be released from the egg sac. Since loose blood is irritating to tissues, this can cause pain. *Mittelschmerz* pain usually lasts only a day or two and may be accompanied by a small amount of vaginal bleeding. Diagnosis is made by finding no other abnormalities during an exam, and by the cyclic nature of the symptoms. No treatment, besides aspirin for pain, if necessary, is required.

☐ *Endometriosis,* which was discussed earlier, is a common cause of pelvic pain. Pain usually comes on with a menstrual period or just before it, and is felt wherever the endometrial patches have attached. Pain also often occurs during sex. Bowel movements may be uncomfortable if the rectum is involved, and severe cramplike pain can arise if the uterus is involved.

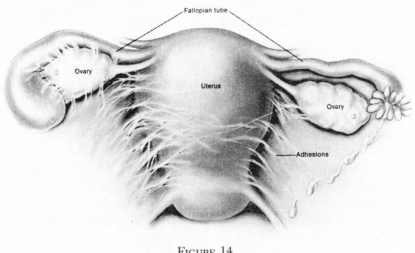

FIGURE 14

Pelvic inflammatory disease
Courtesy of Syntex Laboratories, Inc.

Lower abdominal pain is sometimes due to emotional stress. Diagnosis in these cases is usually done by ruling out physical causes. The treatment would involve emotional support, such as some type of therapy.

The diagnosis of pelvic pain is reached by taking a careful history, by physical examination of the abdomen and the pelvic organs, and then by a group of diagnostic tests. Those that may be of value include an intravenous pyelogram (an x-ray of the kidneys, bladder, and urinary system); barium enema (x-ray of the bowel); small intestine x-ray studies; pelvic sonography (the use of sound waves to construct a picture of the internal organs); and laparoscopy, which is done by inserting a viewing instrument into the abdomen to see what is going on there. Laparoscopy is probably the ultimate diagnostic test for gynecologic problems and is very useful in the diagnosis and management of pelvic pain.

Pelvic pain is common enough so that most women are likely to experience several different types during their menstruating years. Your gynecologist is your best guide to what is significant and what need not worry you. By understanding your anatomy and the potential causes of pain, you can ease your anxiety about what's going on (which, in itself, often diminishes some of the pain) and participate in setting things right again.

ABNORMAL PAP SMEARS

Cancer of the cervix is one of the most serious of all the cancers affecting young women, especially in its potential effect on reproduction. The fact that the cervix is easy to see and easy to get to, unlike most body organs, has enabled truly stunning advances to be made in the treatment and understanding of this disease. It is now known, for example, that outright cancer of the cervix is preceded by earlier, less serious, noncancerous cell changes (known as "dysplasia") and by *carcinoma in situ* (cancer which has not spread). The progression of one form to the next may take a period of years; our ability to recognize the cancer precursors, and to diagnose their presence by the inexpensive and painless test called a "Pap smear," has led to a dramatic reduction in invasive cervical cancer and its death rate. Early recognition and treatment here can also preserve reproductive capacity. In the last twenty years, the incidence of severe invasive cancer of the cervix has decreased about 66 percent. The death rate has dropped 60 percent.

These changing proportions closely parallel the increase in the number of Pap smears being performed. Similar statistics have been reported in many different countries; it is clear that the drops in invasive cancer and deaths are directly related to the increased use of Pap smears.

The American Cancer Society estimates that there will be approximately 16,000 cases of invasive cancer of the cervix diagnosed in the United States this year. But there are about *three times* that number of early *carcinomas in situ*. The cause of cancer of the cervix is, as with most cancers, unknown. However, epidemiologic studies (in which scientists try to find links among large numbers of people with the same particular problem) have identified certain characteristics associated with cervical cancer. By identifying high-risk groups, scientists uncover more clues about the cancer's cause and, at the same time, allow those at risk to be more carefully screened for signs of the disease.

But not all clues reveal usable answers—at least not right away. For example, many investigators have noted that cancer of the cervix is less common among Jewish women. This led some to speculate that sex with a circumcised man might somehow be less of a hazard than sex with an uncircumcised man. Inadequate cleaning of the penis, especially under the foreskin, was then suspected of leading to a concentration of some kind of cancer-causing agent. That theory was undercut, however, by a report from India, in which no difference was found in cervical cancer rates between circumcised Moslems and uncircumcised Hindus. The guessed-at link is still *there*—Jewish women do get less cervical cancer—but doctors just haven't yet figured out *why*.

There are also many studies showing a link between sex and cervical cancer. When many pieces of research agree, chances are good that the apparent connection is a real one. The "why" may be as elusive as ever, though. Many studies show that cervical cancer risk is increased by an early marriage or by having sex at an early age. Some studies suggest that ages fifteen to twenty are the vulnerable time—during which the initial and subsequent sexual encounters somehow predispose a woman to the development of cervical cancer, as much as some thirty years later. Multiple sexual partners, and a history of sexually transmitted diseases, are also associated with a higher risk of cervical cancer. At various times sperm, trichomonas, chlamydia, and herpes have all been under suspicion as cancer triggers. At the present time the condyloma virus, which causes genital warts, looks the most suspicious, but, as yet, this connection also remains unproven.

Table 2 reviews the types of premalignant and malignant conditions in the cervix, their characteristics, and the current treatment. The earliest, and very common, nonmalignant form of this disease is called "mild dysplasia." This may progress to moderate and severe dysplasia, then on to *carcinoma in situ*, and, eventually, to invasive, malignant cancer. The early mild dysplasia can be picked up by the Pap smear, and appropriate treatment may be given with excellent success rates. Even *carcinoma in situ* has an almost 100 percent cure rate. Pap smears are routinely done at the beginning of pregnancy, and many doctors will suggest a Pap smear at checkups to nonpregnant women.

Most women with cancer of the cervix have no symptoms, though occasionally bleeding or staining after sex is an early sign. Pain is not a symptom until the very late stages of cervical cancer. Development of the Pap smear has led to diagnoses long before there are any visible abnormalities of the cervix. This technique was introduced by two scientists, named Papanicolaou (from which "Pap" comes) and Traut, in 1943. A grading system from one to five has been adopted for reporting results of the test. Pap smear Class 1 is negative: All cells are normal. Class 2 shows inflammatory cells, often a sign of infection.

TABLE 2

STAGES OF CERVICAL CANCER

STAGE	Dysplasia	Preinvasive cancer	Invasive cancer			
	Mild Moderate Severe	(*Carcinoma in situ*)	STAGE			
			I	II	III	IV
COMMON TREATMENT	Cryosurgery Cone biopsy Laser surgery	Cone biopsy Laser surgery Cryosurgery Hysterectomy	Radical hysterectomy Radiotherapy	Radiotherapy		
CURE RATES	99%	99%	75%– 80%	50%– 55%	30%– 35%	10%

Class 3 means some suspicious or abnormal cells are present. Classes 4 and 5 mean cancer cells were found (see Table 3).

There is a false-negative rate of as high as 20 percent in the technique itself. This means that, in women who have a cervical abnormality, one time in five the smear doesn't happen to pick up any abnormal cells (so the result was falsely negative, or incorrectly showed no abnormality). That is why Pap smears should be done once a year, even though it can take many years for an early abnormality to progress to cancer.

When a Pap smear comes back positive (meaning it shows abnormal cells), but no suspicious areas are visible to the doctor's naked eye, a colposcopy will probably be done. The colposcope is essentially a magnifying instrument, used to examine the cervix in the doctor's office. A speculum is inserted to hold the vagina open, and the cervix is scanned after it has been stained with a solution that makes the abnormal areas stand out by contrast. Tiny bits of tissue (cervical

TABLE 3

CLASSIFICATION OF PAP SMEARS

CLASS	DEFINITION	CLINICAL FOLLOW-UP
I	Only normal cells	Repeat Pap every year
II	Abnormal cells of type not associated with cancer	Doctor will treat the infection if inflammatory cells present. Pap repeated 3–6-month intervals
III	Cells suspicious for precancer (dysplasia) or cancer	Colposcopy & biopsy. If lesions seen, direct biopsy done. Treatment as in Table I.
IV	Many abnormal cells; high probability of cancer	
V	Cancer cells present	

biopsy) may be taken from any odd-looking areas for study in a lab. The results of these biopsies will usually determine the best treatment approach. Sometimes nothing will be done—mild dysplasias may get better on their own in a few months. Cryosurgery (freezing of the cervix) and laser therapy are treatments for mild forms of the disease. Neither of these treatments impairs fertility in any way.

If the diagnosis isn't clear with the biopsy, further diagnostic procedures may be done. The "cone biopsy" or "conization" is one example. Conization of the cervix involves removing a small cone-shaped piece of tissue from around the opening of the cervix. Cutting out this larger piece of tissue often provides both diagnosis *and* cure. There is enough tissue to almost always reveal the problem, plus the entire abnormality; and most of the potential area for subsequent development of cancer is safely removed. Usually conization does not affect childbearing. In rare cases it may contribute to a condition known as "cervical incompetence." This problem can almost always be treated successfully during pregnancy. The use of colposcopy has eliminated much of the need for cone biopsies, which, however, still remain an important tool in evaluating the extent of and treating cervical disease.

Guidelines for treating *carcinoma in situ* are shown in the following options.

- If a young woman still wants to have children, and the cancer is truly *in situ* (has not spread), it can be treated by a cone biopsy. This will remove 90 percent of the potential cancer-producing area, but still allows the woman to conceive and carry a child. However, Pap smears at least twice a year as follow-ups are required to keep a close watch on the condition.
- If the woman has no desire for more children, and if there is no strong emotional reason for preserving menstrual function, a hysterectomy (removal of the uterus) can be done. There is no reason, however, to remove the ovaries.
- If the woman is pregnant when diagnosed, the pregnancy is allowed to continue. A cone biopsy may be done safely during the pregnancy for both diagnostic and therapeutic purposes.

Cervical cancer in its most severe form—invasive cancer—must be treated by an operation called a "radical hysterectomy." This involves the removal of the uterus, the ovaries, and the surrounding pelvic tissue, including the lymph nodes that drain the area. The most extensive cancers may also be treated with radiation therapy, as outlined in Table 2.

The five-year survival rate for cancer of the cervix depends on the stage of the disease when it is found. Remember, however, that the vast majority of cervical cancers are caught early, when they are *highly* curable and have little or no impact on fertility. The key to that kind of early diagnosis and happy outcome is as simple as the routine Pap smear.

This list of problem after problem may make even the least anxious woman feel a twinge of "there are so many things that can go wrong!" But common as many of these conditions are, any one woman is likely to experience only a few, at most. And the vast majority of these conditions have little or no impact on your future fertility—especially if they're caught and treated early. And that's exactly the point: The more you know about what might go wrong, the easier it is to avoid problems altogether, or at least minimize their effects on your body.

PART III

Planning and Adjusting to Your Pregnancy

Introduction

The time a couple spends planning for a pregnancy can be almost as exciting as the period of gestation itself. It has its own unique challenges, its own sense of specialness. It is a time to prepare your body, your relationship with your partner, your work life—in short, to put your life in order so that the upcoming change from couple to family will be as smooth and satisfying as you can make it.

To help you achieve this goal, I'll take you through some of the factors it is important to consider at this time. And there are quite a few areas that demand attention! For example, if you would like to work throughout your pregnancy, what do you need to know about the impact of your job on both your body and that of your developing fetus? And what about the reverse—will your pregnancy affect your ability to do your job? Are you exposed to any chemicals at work, or at home, or do you take any medications your doctor should know about in helping you plan for a healthy conception? How different is it to have a baby when you're over thirty? Should you start to eat differently, change the type of exercise you do? As for genetic counseling before pregnancy, how does a woman or her partner even know whether or not it's necessary for them? Some of the facts in this section will probably surprise you.

Finally, there's a "Prepregnancy Checklist," a kind of at-a-glance, sum-up reminder of all the things you should be planning to do—from getting your teeth cleaned to quitting smoking, seeing your gynecologist, and gaining or losing weight—in the months before the planning stages of a healthy pregnancy draw to a close and the time to actually try for pregnancy begins.

If you've been taking good care of your health and any health problems as they arise, you've already done much to increase the chances of health for your future children. Your obstetrician will work with you once you become pregnant, perhaps suggesting various tests to monitor the health of your fetus, such as blood tests, ultrasound, and amniocentesis, to do as much as possible to ensure that those good odds continue. (The various tests are discussed in Chapter 20, "Prenatal Testing.")

Adjusting to Pregnancy

No matter how much you want a child, you are bound to have some worries and conflicting emotions once you find out you actually are pregnant. Changing the structure of a family—and that's exactly what the birth of a child does—always requires some adjustment. Conflicting emotions may be even greater for a woman having a child at a later age. After investing so much time in building a career, a relationship, an entire life that doesn't contain a child, it's normal to feel torn at the thought of what might have to be given up, at the changes you will have to make.

Many women are facing similar dilemmas, as more and more professional women in their thirties start families. During the decade of the 1970s, the number of thirty-five- to thirty-nine-year-old college graduates who were first-time mothers nearly doubled.

"It's very exciting, and not just a little frightening," I was told by Martha, a thirty-four-year-old physician who was pregnant with her first child. "I'm used to scheduling my time in a logical and disciplined manner, knowing exactly what's required of me. But I can't yet see exactly how my life will be affected by this new human being. For the first time, I can't plan for every minute. I just have to wait and see."

While you can't plan exactly how a baby will affect your life and work, that doesn't mean you can't plan at all. You can make some basic decisions that will work with your life and your needs and have some flexibility built in so they can give with the unforeseen. Some women plan to work full time after having a child. Others decide they'll resolve the tug between the need for both babies and work by having a part-time job. Still others think they will simply put their careers on hold for a while. But if you survey a few friends who have been in this position, you may realize that even the best-laid plans sometimes take a 180-degree turn: The woman who was convinced that staying home with an infant for six months would drive her batty couldn't drag herself away from her baby for a year. And the mother who thought it would be a nice change to stay out of the office rat race for a while, finds herself hungering for those challenges her years on the job trained her to meet. It's not a bad idea, then, to make a second or even a third backup plan so, whichever one ends up seeming right, some planning will already have gone into it. By being sensitive to, and honest about, your own feelings and the needs of your family, and by talking things over with your partner, you should be able to make decisions that are right for you and your family. And if one decision doesn't work, plans can always be scrapped, and a new strategy tried.

Sally, a thirty-two-year-old freelance writer, found that she gradually settled into a routine that accommodated both her child's needs and her work. "It took some experimentation, and I had to train myself to keep my attention on my writing when my daughter was in the next room. But just as I never could have foreseen all the difficulties, I was also enchanted by the unexpected rewards," she told me.

Obviously, your relationship with your partner also undergoes changes when you have a baby. If you've been a couple for a long time, you've probably developed daily routines and leisure activities that are comfortable and satisfying. Change, even longed-for change, can present a difficult challenge. It also can end up, as it does in the vast majority of cases, adding richness and intensity to your feelings for each other. Pregnancy and childbirth are exciting and immensely rewarding events. Age should not prevent you from being able to have a child safely and happily. Your obstetrician, your partner, and your friends are all there to help. Use them to air your fears, lean on when you need them, and, finally, to share with you the joys of having a child.

9

The Working Woman
and Pregnancy

Over the past ten years, the number of women in professional oc-
cupations has increased by nearly 60 percent. The number holding
managerial positions has more than doubled. The number of women
in sales, service, and clerical jobs has also increased. The proportion
of women obtaining professional degrees has increased dramatically,
especially in such fields as medicine, dentistry, law, optometry, and
theology. In some of these areas the number of women graduates has
increased tenfold! And behind these impressive statistics are creative,
intelligent, ambitious women who also plan to be mothers.

Today nearly half of all children under the age of six have working
mothers. Over 60 percent of kids six to seventeen also have mothers
who work. Why have women sought employment outside the home
in such dramatic proportions? One reason is that two-wage-earner
families have become necessary in some parts of the country to maintain even an average standard of living. Sometimes women begin to
work for special projects—a child's college education, or buying a
home—and never stop. One in five American children lives *only* with
the mother, who must work to support them. Still other women need
the feelings of achievement and social contacts they gain from paid
employment. Some find the very special responsibilities of child care
overwhelming without the balancing factor of work. Finally, there are
many well-educated women who possess the abilities for a professional
career and, quite simply, want to achieve that status without giving
up the option of having a family.

The life of the working woman and mother involves considerable compromise. There must be, to keep the family, the job, and herself going. Sometimes it is very difficult to excel in a career and, at the same time, raise a family well. As one thirty-seven-year-old working mother of three explained it, "I'm always torn. When I'm at the office, I worry about the kids at home. When I'm with them, something left undone at work nags at me. But then I remind myself that all mothers worry about their children, and all professionals feel there's more work to do than time to do it. I'm glad I have the chance to do both."

There are sacrifices involved in juggling work and home responsibilities. Although more women than ever are working, often shouldering the same responsibilities as men, most mothers still carry the burden of managing the household and raising the children. A working wife enjoys substantially less leisure time and sleep than her spouse. Women who work and are married find very little time in the course of the day to just relax and unwind. In addition, the ingrained cultural ideals about the way children are supposed to be raised remain alive, leading to feelings of guilt and inadequacy on the part of some working women. Psychiatrists and pediatricians, sometimes inadvertently, tend to increase the guilt with their recommendations of optimal times to work and biases about the joys of motherhood and mothers in general.

Eventually, all this can take its toll. Many talented and self-confident women who began climbing the corporate ladder in the 1970s are now dropping out, having decided they couldn't do both. It has nothing to do with their willingness to work hard or their abilities. It has a lot to do with the high standards they set for *every* aspect of their lives. Says one mother of two preschoolers, "I could not be an excellent bank executive *and* an excellent mother. I chose to concentrate on one thing for now: my kids. In a few years, when they're in school full time, I want to go back to work. For now, I'm happier knowing I'm at least doing one thing to the best of my ability."

Other women try to work it out differently. "Housekeepers and husbands are the key," one laughingly told me. "Seriously, though, you can't do it all yourself. And you shouldn't feel guilty for that either. I think my family is maybe even happier, more secure, because the responsibility is spread out, than they would be in a more traditional setup."

Another category of working mother today is the single mother. Whether they're divorced or widowed, life for these women is much more difficult because they must make all the decisions and arrangements alone. There is also a new group, unmarried women who have chosen to have their children alone. The number of single women giving birth rose 20 percent between 1970 and 1981. Of course, this figure also includes many women who were not planning to become mothers but decided not to have abortions. However, the middle-class, career-conscious, unmarried mother-by-choice has taken over an increasing share of this number.

PLANNING YOUR FAMILY

There is no such thing as a totally convenient time to have a child. It used to be that couples fresh out of high school or college would have babies at once. Now many men and women are hesitating, waiting longer to get married and have their children. While this can then make the change from couple to family a bigger step, there are advantages to waiting.

A working couple, by delaying parenting, is usually in a stronger financial position to weather the costs of children and child care. Job advancement usually means larger salaries, so help from housekeepers and day care centers can be more easily afforded. Delayed childbearing also helps ease some psychological strains of balancing this often difficult money situation.

Maturity is a big bonus that can make some of the work-versus-motherhood struggles easier. Once your reputation has been established, the work load may decrease naturally, or it may be easier to do it by choice. It becomes less necessary to prove yourself to your employer or colleagues. The longer a woman works, the more likely it is that her employer has a vested interest in keeping her. Seniority may even win special concessions such as maternity leaves, more flexible working hours, and variable vacations.

Delayed parenthood also gives women time to forge a solid professional identity—build up a work track record and achieve promotions. Once in this position, even if they take a few years off to have children, women are likely to have an easier time coming back into the professional arena.

More and more working couples are scaling down their family size. The birthrate in this country today is less than half of that in the late 1950s, when it reached a record high. The American family now averages less than two children; many families stop at one. This may be especially appealing to those trying to juggle a career and motherhood. One such woman says, "I grew up in a family of five. Mom stayed home to raise us. I always pictured having a big family, and worried about 'deprived' only children. But my Samantha gets more attention from us than I could from my parents; and she has lots of friends and her cousins to relate to. She's thriving as an only child."

If you want more than one child, spacing the children two to three years apart seems to be best. This is good medically, and psychologically reduces the strain on parents and the first-born child. By age three, a child has become slightly more independent and is less likely to resent the intrusion of the new baby. Also, by this time the older child is usually more manageable, out of diapers, and amenable to reasoning. However, there is no one best spacing time for all families. Many couples I know have children less than two and a half years apart; and, of course, women who have waited until their late thirties may not have the fertile time to wait three years between children.

WORKING WHILE PREGNANT

Over one million women, working in a wide variety of jobs, become pregnant each year. Many will work until just before delivery and return to work within weeks after birth. Because of this trend we must examine the question: Is it safe for pregnant women to work?

A pregnant working woman should discuss her own particular job situation and conditions with her physician. Basically, if you are a normal, healthy woman with an uncomplicated pregnancy and a normally developing fetus, you may work at no increased risk right up to when labor begins. You may also resume working several weeks after giving birth. But if your job is strenuous and requires a lot of standing or walking, your physician may ask you to cut back on your work hours and, perhaps, to stop working a few weeks before delivery.

Some job situations may expose you to work conditions that could be harmful to you or your baby. (These are discussed at the end of the chapter.) In those cases you may have to be transferred to another job, or stop working. Women with a history of certain maternal problems—a history of miscarriages or premature births—or who are carrying twins, may be advised to stop working.

The decision to continue working during pregnancy will depend on your preference, overall health, how your pregnancy is progressing, your age, and any problems you may have had during past pregnancies. The type of work you do, how many hours you work, and any job-related threats to you or your fetus should also be considered.

Your doctor's advice may vary during the course of pregnancy, depending on changes in your condition, your job, or your lifestyle. Your pregnancy may also lead to disabilities that prevent you from performing your usual duties. Such disability usually falls into one of three categories:

1. Disability due to the pregnancy itself. Some women have pregnancy-related side effects such as nausea, vomiting, indigestion, dizziness, swollen legs and ankles—all of which may cause temporary problems while working. Your doctor will reevaluate these problems at regular intervals, giving you guidelines each time.
2. Disability from a complication of pregnancy. Most serious complications—infection, bleeding, rupture of the amniotic sac—may make you physically unable to continue working. Medical conditions you had before becoming pregnant, such as heart disease, diabetes, or high blood pressure, may also make working while pregnant more risky.
3. Disability related to the job. Some disabilities may be work-related, such as exposure to toxic substances or strenuous labor.

If your doctor decides that your pregnancy is disabling, he or she can verify to your employer that you are eligible for any disability compensation the company offers. On the other hand, if your doctor says you are able to keep working, your employer may request a letter written by your doctor stating so.

Maternity policies vary from job to job. Only about 40 percent of employed women in the United States are entitled to a paid six-week disability leave for childbirth. Others are forced to use sick leave or vacation time, or take time off without pay. The Pregnancy Discrimination Act passed by Congress in 1978 requires employers who offer medical disability to treat pregnancy-related disabilities in the same manner as all others. This means that, if you are temporarily unable to work because of pregnancy, your employer must give you the same rights as other employees temporarily disabled by illness or accident. If your employer regularly assigns lighter work to other partially disabled workers, the same must be done for you. Unfortunately, many employers offer no disability benefits at all and, therefore, are not obliged to provide maternity leave. If no disability plan is offered where you work you may qualify for temporary disability benefits from your state. Your local unemployment office is the best place to find out about state benefits and how you may qualify.

Disability related to job exposure is often hard to establish. There is still much to be learned about the effects on pregnancy of toxic substances, physical strains, stress, and other possible health threats the working woman may encounter. The few studies that have been done have produced conflicting results. Until more is known, common sense on your part and a knowledge of established hazards on your doctor's is the best way to minimize risks involved in working during pregnancy.

HAZARDS ON THE JOB

Exposure of pregnant women to certain chemicals and substances is known to increase the likelihood of fetal abnormalities, miscarriages, premature birth, and problems that appear later in the baby's life. In such cases you may have to be transferred to another job or stop working. A few examples follow, and a more complete listing of potentially hazardous materials women may encounter both on and off the job is included in Chapter 13, "Environmental Hazards to Pregnancy."

☐ *Metals* have been linked to stillbirths, mental retardation, some birth defects, and miscarriage. Industries in which the risk of metal poisoning is greatest, especially exposure to "heavy" metals such as lead and mercury, are lead smelting, battery manufacturing, paint manufacturing, painting, printing, ceramics, pottery glazing, and glass manufacturing. Toll booth attendants and others who work on heavily traveled roads may have high levels of lead in their blood. Mercury vapors may be inhaled in the workplaces of dentists, dental hygienists, technicians, and laboratory workers.

☐ *Radiation* emitted by x-rays can harm the fetus, since high levels of radiation are suspected of causing genetic damage, miscarriage, cancer, and some birth defects. Women with the greatest risk of radiation exposure are x-ray technicians and some researchers who use radioisotopes. If you are planning a pregnancy and are exposed to radiation in a medical or industrial setting, you should have monthly readings of the amount of radiation you've been exposed to. The safe limit commonly cited for radiation exposure during the course of pregnancy is 10 rads. Diagnostic x-rays using less than 10 rads have little or no risk. Radiation from microwave ovens, video display terminals, and television sets has not been found to pose any health hazard during pregnancy, since these are a different, "nonionizing," form of radiation.

☐ *Anaesthetic gases*   seem to expose women working in an operating room or a dentist's office to a greater risk of miscarriage and of bearing babies with birth defects.

☐ *Heavy physical work*   such as having to lift heavy things, climb many stairs, or do other work requiring a great use of energy causes discomfort in some women during pregnancy. The first few months may bring periods of dizziness and fatigue, which can increase the risk of accidents. Toward the end of pregnancy women may find their balance is "off" and they have become more vulnerable to falling.

Before you accept a job, find out from the employer if you may be exposed to toxic substances, chemicals, or radiation. Talk to the personnel officer about maternity benefits and disability coverage. If you work while pregnant, take good care of yourself and have regular checkups. If possible, keep some nourishing snacks (fruit, nuts) near your work station, and try to rest during breaks. If you have any questions about what is safe, ask your doctor.

At home, housework and care of other children does not stop during pregnancy. These can also be strenuous. You may need to share more responsibilities with your partner or others to ensure that you get enough rest. Careful planning and sufficient sleep become very important, to avoid too much stress and strain. It is even more important, if you are working, to maintain the overall healthy-pregnancy lifestyle that this book is all about.

10

Pregnancy After Thirty

Many more women today are having their first child after age thirty. Between 1970 and 1979 the rate of women having children between ages thirty and forty-four rose about 66 percent. In 1979, nearly 20 percent of children born to thirty-four-year-old women were first children—double the percentage of just ten years before. And in the twelve-month period ending in June 1984, the birthrate for women aged thirty to thirty-four rose to 72.2 per 1,000 women—compared with 56.4 per 1,000 women in 1976. Most of these women were college graduates and professionals who wanted to establish their careers before starting to raise families.

Women who are considering having children in their thirties or forties often have many questions and concerns, about their ability to conceive in the first place, the ability of their bodies to carry and deliver a baby, about the health of a child born to an "older" woman. Worries like these are not entirely unwarranted, but it is important to understand that there's nothing magic about thirty. People age bit by bit, not all at once.

We also age unequally. Take two thirty-year-olds and stand them side by side. Now add a pair of forty-year-olds to the lineup. If you then brought in someone from a soundproof booth and asked them to tell you how old your four women were, chances are they'd pick a range—maybe twenty-five to forty-five. And for all intents and purposes, they might be just about right. A "young" forty-year-old might well have no more problems with a pregnancy than an "old" twenty-five-year-old. The woman of forty might be slim, well muscled, have lots of stamina and energy, eat and sleep healthily, forgo smoking, and drink only an occasional glass of wine. Her younger counterpart might be plump, smoke like a chimney, and pant breathlessly after trudging up one flight of steps. Exaggerated, obviously, but you get the point. Age is only one of the factors involved in a healthy pregnancy. Even problems that are age-linked can be minimized by working closely—right from the start of your planning stage—with your obstetrician.

AGE AND FERTILITY

It's hard to say precisely how age will affect any one woman's ability to conceive. As you will see from the in-depth chapter on fertility problems, the causes of infertility—which I will define here as the inability of a couple to produce a child—are multiple and complex. Many students have tried to examine the precise relationship of infertility and maternal age. But most have been criticized by experts in the field for not "controlling for," or taking into account, enough of the possible variables—factors like the health of the father, and the number of menstrual cycles the study looked at.

In order to try to eliminate these confounding variables, a now-classic French study looked at the success of artificial insemination (in which donor sperm are deposited at the top of a woman's vagina) in women who had never conceived, and whose husbands had produced no sperm. The results showed a slight but significant decrease in the conception rate starting at age thirty and becoming more marked after age thirty-five. Even this study has been criticized for not accounting for the differences between natural and artificial insemination and between childless women and those who already had children. Still, along with all the other studies, the French report does seem to indicate that there is a slight but constant fall in fertility as women get older.

One reason for this may be that the frequency of ovulation is likely to drop as a woman approaches menopause. Born with about one million eggs, she will have about 500,000 healthy eggs remaining at puberty. Each month fifty or so of these eggs will ripen in preparation for ovulation. But within a few days, most of these will have degenerated, usually leaving only one ripe egg ready for release.

Since your ovaries hold fewer eggs as you grow older, you may not be ovulating every month, even though you have a menstrual period. This could mean that you might have to spend several months trying to conceive before the timing is just right and you become pregnant.

As usual, though, that's not the only factor. How often you have sex, your partner's health, your own gynecologic history, all will have an impact. And as you get older, you're more likely to have encountered some of the hazards that can affect fertility, such as pelvic infections from sexually transmitted diseases, endometriosis (growth outside the uterus of the tissue that normally lines it), fibroids (noncancerous tumors in the uterine wall), and the effects of other pregnancies on your body.

Since 80 percent of all couples conceive within twelve months of starting to try, about a year's trying is recommended before a couple should seek a full-scale infertility investigation. However, if you're over thirty, you might want to seek professional advice after six months, simply because you have a shorter period of fertility ahead. For those couples found to have a problem, new diagnostic and treatment strategies are enabling many couples who had previously not been able to procreate to have children.

PREGNANCY AND DELIVERY AFTER THIRTY

Other problems besides difficulty with conception may also increase slightly after thirty. Again, it's difficult to say just how much higher the chances of, for example, a miscarriage after thirty really are. For one thing, now we can diagnose pregnancy so much earlier than ever before—as early as nine days after conception, even before a period is missed—that what appears to be a higher miscarriage rate may only be a more accurate counting of miscarriages that were occurring all along. New figures are leading experts to suspect that nearly half of all fertilized eggs may abort spontaneously, without the woman's even knowing that she became pregnant. It's the body's way of quickly and easily dealing with a defective pregnancy, without disturbing the rhythm of the menstrual cycle.

Since women aren't always aware when they've had a spontaneous abortion, it's impossible to determine exactly how much more frequently this occurs in older women. In general, miscarriage is recognizable in about 15 percent of all pregnancies. It seems slightly more frequent in women over thirty, but not enough so to become a major problem. In women over thirty-five the proportion of stillbirths (babies born dead) is slightly higher than in women aged twenty to thirty. The proportion of low-birth-weight babies is also slightly higher for women over thirty-five. The proportion of women having cesarean sections for delivery is again slightly higher for women having their first child after thirty-five. One factor for this last may be, of course, that many obstetricians are quicker to opt for surgery for an older mother over a more "wait and see" approach at delivery.

BIRTH DEFECTS

This is often a major concern to older women considering pregnancy. It should be reassuring to know that most children in the United States are born healthy and normal. The cause of birth defects isn't always known, though age is a factor in some cases, as are heredity and environmental exposures. Certain couples do have a greater than normal chance of having a child born with a physical abnormality. However, while the likelihood of some problems does increase with age, it remains low well into the thirties.

As with other age-tied problems, there's no abrupt jump in the rate of birth defects as a couple gets older. For example, the chances of having a child with Down's syndrome—a condition involving many mental and physical abnormalities—increase steadily as the mother ages. It is the only clearly age-related birth defect. Only one in 1,600 children born to mothers in their early twenties would be expected to have this problem. On the other hand, Down's syndrome occurs in one of 365 children born to women at the age of thirty-five. At age forty the risk is one in 100; and at forty-five it's one in 32. Striking as this increased risk is, you should note that even at forty a woman has a 99 percent chance of *not* having a baby with Down's syndrome; even at forty-five she has a 97 percent chance.

Identifying your dangers of having a child with a birth defect is one of the main reasons to start working closely with your obstetrician in planning a pregnancy, before you even start trying to get pregnant. Couples in the high-risk groups, because of age or other factors, can still have normal, healthy children. And the doctor can increase the chances of that happening. But the couple needs to be well-informed about the risks that apply to them, and discuss their plans and any known problems with their obstetrician, so that medical supervision can be provided.

If you are thirty-five or over, already have a child with birth defects, or have a family history of genetic disorders or a personal history of miscarriages or stillbirths, your obstetrician may recommend genetic counseling. (See Chapter 14, "Genetic Counseling.") This will allow you to assess your risks and make an informed decision about having a child. Such counseling is done by doctors, nurses, or health educators with special training in genetics. They can give you important information based on your family history, personal history, and sometimes a physical exam and laboratory tests.

Relying on the genetic counseling information obtained from these specialists and the guidance of your obstetrician, you can then do everything possible to ensure a healthy pregnancy and birth. Health care before conception (preconceptual care) is especially necessary for women over thirty. The first eight weeks or so of pregnancy—when many women don't even know yet whether they are pregnant—are some of the most important for the baby. This is, for one example, the time the organs are being formed; women particularly concerned about these early weeks might want to consider pregnancy testing at the earliest possible time. About three and a half weeks after the last menstrual period, for a woman with a twenty-eight-day cycle, isn't too soon for fast new over-the-counter tests that have just come on the market. (See Chapter 16, "Becoming Pregnant and Early Pregnancy," for more about pregnancy tests.)

11

Nutrition in Pregnancy

During pregnancy the mother is the sole source of all the nutrients her fetus needs for growth and development. If this supply is too low, fetal growth may be affected—an infant may be born with a condition known as "intrauterine growth retardation" (IUGR). These small babies may have problems after birth; the dramatic result of severe food deprivation has been graphically demonstrated during famines in various areas of the world. During famine periods the average birth weight falls as much as 10 percent.

But IUGR doesn't happen only in remote, third-world countries. Poor women in this country whose food supply is limited and very underweight women are also at risk. Maternal malnutrition also exists among pregnant adolescents and, surprisingly, affluent women who limit their food intake for some reason such as weight control or fad diets. Also, excessive physical activity can use up so much of the mother's energy intake as possibly to deprive the fetus of needed calories for growth. Babies born in developing countries during the months of heavy agricultural labor are lower in birth weight than babies born at other times of the year. While the food supply of these active pregnant women may not be limited, their nutritional needs may differ from those of the sedentary pregnant woman. I will consider the special needs of the active pregnant woman after my general guidelines for eating during pregnancy.

Good maternal nutrition should begin even before you become pregnant. Women who start off too thin are more likely to deliver small babies even if they eat right and gain weight normally during pregnancy. Women who are too fat when they conceive are more likely to have difficulties with delivery and to develop high blood pressure. However, pregnancy is *not* a time to diet. Along with depriving the fetus of the critical nutritional support it needs, extreme dieting, with the breakdown of fat that occurs, can release toxic substances called "ketone bodies" that could harm the fetus.

BASIC PRINCIPLES OF NUTRITION IN PREGNANCY

☐ *Caloric intake and weight gain.* The total number of calories consumed appears to be the single most important nutritional factor affecting infant birth weight. But "eating for two"—even for one and a half—is out. A typical sedentary pregnancy requires about 300 extra calories per day, assuming that you maintain your normal level of activity. Active pregnant woman need more. That is only the amount in one generous scoop of ice cream; you obviously can't eat everything in sight. And you can't even just go for that ice cream every day. You have to spend those added extra calories wisely, on the extra nutrients your baby needs: extra protein, calcium, iron, and B vitamins.

Twenty-four to twenty-six pounds is considered the appropriate amount of weight to gain during the average pregnancy. But the rate of gain is as important as the total amount. A pound and a half to three pounds during the entire first three months, and one pound every nine days thereafter, is average. The quickest weight gain occurs in the last three months, when the fetus is growing quickly (see Figure 15).

A total weight gain of about 24 pounds will break down the following way. The baby will weigh about 7½ pounds at birth, the placenta 1½ pounds, the amniotic fluid 2 pounds, an increase in the size of the uterus 2 pounds, increase in breast size 1 pound. Fat and water in the maternal tissues weigh about 6–10 pounds, and the increase in the mother's blood volume is 4 pounds. A week or two after the baby is born you will have lost 18 to 20 pounds. Within four months most women will have lost the remainder of the pounds if they are not breastfeeding.

Women who start out underweight should gain about 30 pounds, or about 6 over the normal 24. A weight gain of greater than 30 pounds is not recommended, no matter how thin a woman is when she conceives. Excessive weight gain may result in permanent obesity, with its resulting complications of high blood pressure, diabetes, and heart disease. Although many women who gain excessive weight during pregnancy *do* lose it after delivery, too many women retain the excess.

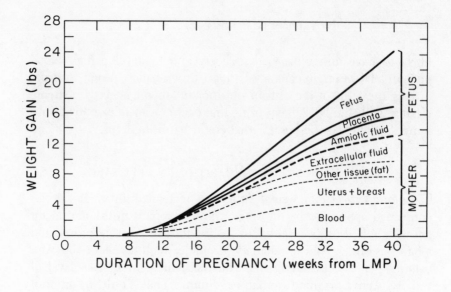

FIGURE 15

Weight gain in pregnancy. A gain of twenty-five pounds is divided on the right of the chart into fetal and maternal components.

Nutrition in pregnancy, therefore, is a delicate balance of taking in the right nutrients without overdoing the calories. Even women with minimal willpower find the idea of doing right by the baby a strong source of motivation to keep them eating right but without dieting.

☐ *Protein.* An increase of 30 grams of protein per day is recommended for pregnancy. This makes the total intake 75 to 100 grams of protein per day; that should be about 12 percent of total calories. Most protein-containing foods are also excellent sources of many vitamins and minerals essential for the fetus, such as iron, vitamin B_6, and zinc. In addition to the milk products every pregnant woman should have, you need at least three servings a day of either meat, fish, poultry, or eggs.

There is no evidence that eating more than 100 grams of protein per day is of any value. A high-protein, low-calorie diet is *not* desirable during pregnancy. You need the steady supply of energy which can be provided best by carbohydrates.

In recent years vegetarian diets, which exclude some or all animal proteins, have become quite popular. These diets can provide adequate nutrition, but pregnant vegetarians need to be even more careful about food selection than the meat-eating pregnant woman. Lacto-ovo vegetarian diets (those which include dairy products and/or eggs) easily provide all the nutrients needed for pregnancy. But if all animal protein sources are avoided, it's hard to get enough vitamin B_{12} and zinc, iron, calcium, vitamin D, and riboflavin into your meals. If vegetable protein is used to meet the day's requirements, the essential amino acids in the various foods must be properly balanced so the protein intake becomes "complete" in terms of the body's needs. This is achieved by combining grains with beans or nuts, or combining any of these with dairy products in the same meal. Due to the low fat and high bulk of vegetarian foods, pregnant women may have trouble consuming enough calories. Vitamin and mineral supplements are generally recommended, and added vegetable oils and fats may be encouraged if there is too little fuel in the diet otherwise.

☐ *Iron.*   Extra iron is needed during pregnancy for the additional red blood cells the mother produces and for the fetus to produce its own entire blood supply. About 800 milligrams of iron is needed to accomplish this during the second half of pregnancy. This comes to about 5 to 6 milligrams daily, which many women's bodies cannot provide for the fetus without depleting their own stores. Therefore, a daily supplement providing 30 to 60 milligrams of elemental iron is recommended for all pregnant women. Folic acid may also be given as a supplement, since pregnancy doubles your folic acid requirement and helps iron metabolism.

Good food sources of iron include dried fruits, liver, kidneys, prune juice, and dried beans. The type of food selected not only influences the amount of iron you get, it also influences the amount of iron that can be absorbed by your body. Some foods enhance iron absorption, whereas others inhibit it. Animal proteins and vitamin C (ascorbic acid) enhance iron absorption. Tea and milk reduce this absorption and should be avoided at meals, especially when good iron sources are consumed. (Cast iron pans may provide significant amounts of iron, particularly if acidic foods like spaghetti sauce are cooked in them.)

A part of your prepregnancy counseling will include a blood count to rule out the presence of anemia and your physician's prescription for an extra iron supplement if a deficiency is found. If you start a pregnancy iron-depleted or develop anemia during pregnancy, larger doses of iron will be required. If you find yourself constantly overtired, ask your physician to check your iron status an extra time.

☐ *Calcium.* A daily intake of 1,200 milligrams of calcium is recommended during pregnancy to provide the extra 30 grams of calcium required to build your baby's bones. If you don't like milk, you don't have to drink it. Milk products like cheese, yogurt, and cottage cheese are equally good sources of calcium. Whole, skim, or powdered milk can be added to soups and baked goods, even whipped into potatoes. Broccoli, spinach, kale, and mustard greens also supply calcium, but the calcium from vegetables is less easily absorbed by the body.

Four cups—one quart—of yogurt or milk supply the daily recommended amount of calcium. One and a half ounces of cheddar cheese, or one and three-quarters cups of ice cream, or two cups of cottage cheese have the calcium in one cup of milk. If you cannot drink regular milk because you can't digest milk sugar (a common condition, called "lactose intolerance") you should have no trouble with hard, unprocessed cheeses like cheddar or Swiss, and you may be able to handle cultured milk products like yogurt and buttermilk.

☐ *Sodium.* There is an increase in the total amount of water retained in a pregnant woman's body. To keep her chemical balance, she needs to increase the total amount of body sodium—about 22 grams extra.

In the past, salt was forbidden to pregnant women and diuretic ("water") pills were prescribed whenever fluid accumulation occurred. It used to be thought that a high salt intake could cause a serious condition known as "toxemia of pregnancy," and this condition could be treated with salt restriction and diuretics. We now know that neither of these theories is true. In fact, toxemic women have too *little* total body water and salt. Diuretics should not be used in pregnancy unless prescribed by your physician in *very special* cases.

You should salt your foods to taste. A diet based on whole, natural foods can be safely salted within reason. Processed foods are usually heavily preseasoned with salt and should be eaten in moderation, without additional salting.

☐ *Other nutrients.* The body's dietary need for folic acid is increased during pregnancy to support the growth of the fetus. Many vitamin supplements for pregnant women now contain folic acid. (Most doctors will prescribe prenatal vitamins.) Foods rich in folic acid include eggs, leafy vegetables, oranges, whole grain cereals, and wheat germ. The refinement of grains removes many nutrients normally found in wheat germ and bran; zinc, vitamin B_6, magnesium, and vitamin E are of particular concern because these nutrients are not put back during the enrichment process. Whole grain cereals should be included in meals to assure adequate levels of these nutrients and of fiber, which adds bulk and aids bowel function.

☐ *Nutritional needs during breastfeeding.* If you plan to nurse you should know that your nutritional needs are even greater during lactation than during pregnancy. A nursing mother has to produce almost a quart of milk a day to satisfy her tiny, but hungry, baby! To do this she may need close to an extra 1,000 calories a day above her pre-pregnancy diet. These calories should be spent on an extra 40 grams of protein, at least a quart of milk daily, and additional eggs, cheese, liver, and vegetables.

EATING FOR ACTIVE PREGNANT WOMEN

Based on our knowledge of the nutritional needs of pregnancy and of strenuous exercise, we can make some general recommendations for women who exercise during pregnancy.

The additional pregnancy allowance of 300 calories per day provides only for the increased needs of the sedentary pregnant woman. The amount a pregnant woman who exercises should add to this depends, of course, on how much exercise she is getting. Therefore, it is impossible to make a specific recommendation. As a broad suggestion, however, 500 additional calories may be adequate for women who maintain a thirty-minute daily exercise program during pregnancy. If the rate of weight gain begins to fall below normal at any stage, additional calories should be consumed.

If the active pregnant woman is alert to her appetite, she may be able to adjust her food intake to match her physical needs. A diet high in complex carbohydrates is also advised, since carbohydrates best replace muscle glycogen burned during exercise.

Pregnancy increases the need for protein; physical activity may do so as well. However, since the usual protein consumption in the United States is well above the requirement for pregnancy, it probably also covers the additional needs of exercise. In general, the physically active pregnant woman's diet should be about 12 percent protein. If she consumes 2,300 calories a day, about 69 grams should be protein. A woman taking in 3,000 calories a day would need about 90 grams of protein.

The iron needs of all pregnant women are similar, since exercise does not appear to increase the need for iron. But a pregnant woman starting an exercise program would have greater iron needs, to accommodate the blood volume expansion associated with training. However, taking up strenuous exercise during pregnancy is *not* recommended. The requirements of the training program on top of the developing pregnancy may simply be too much for the body to take at once without risking health.

Physically active pregnant women need to drink lots of water in order to replace that depleted during exercise. Taking care to drink extra fluids—and plain water is best—is important to maintain adequate hydration.

Sodium sweated off during exercise also has to be replaced. Although most pregnant women will take in more than enough salt, the physically active pregnant woman may risk sodium depletion if her exercise is vigorous and her sodium intake low. Especially when outdoor exercise in hot weather is prolonged (*not* a good idea anyway), all women should eat extra amounts of salty foods. Table 4 summarizes the various nutritional needs of active pregnant, active nonpregnant, and nonpregnant women.

In summary, energy is the major nutritional need of the physically active pregnant woman. If you get enough total calories, most of the other nutritional requirements will be satisfied, as long as you try to eat a wide variety of foods and keep empty "junk" calories to a minimum. The athletic woman is urged to eat according to her appetite and to double-check the accuracy of this approach by tracking weight gain carefully. I advise these athletic women to buy a good scale and weigh themselves weekly. If the rate of gain deviates from the normal range at any time, calories should be adjusted to get you back on your food track.

TABLE 4

Comparison Summary of Nutritional Needs

	ACTIVE WOMEN	PREGNANT NONACTIVE WOMEN	PREGNANT ACTIVE WOMEN
CALORIES	1. Increase to energy needs 2. Complex carbohydrates important	1. Increase 300 cal/day 2. Increase protein sources	1. Increase 300 cal/day + increase to energy (200–300 cal/day additional) 2. Weight gain is good guide 3. Proteins & carbohydrates
PROTEINS	Normal percentage of calories	Increase to 75 g/day	12% of calories (75–90 g/day)
IRON	1. No increase required after training completed 2. Increase during training	Increase 30–60 mg/day	Increase 30–60 mg/day in trained pregnant women
WATER	During exercise 10–12 glasses of fluids per day	1. Increase fluids to thirst 2. Lactation (one quart extra/day)	1. 8–12 glasses extra water during exercise 2. Increase during heat
SODIUM (SALT)	Increased needs, especially in hot weather	Salt to taste	Increased needs, especially in hot weather
CALCIUM	Retention higher with activity resulting in increased bone density; no additional requirement	Additional 30 g required during pregnancy. Daily 1200 mg calcium	Same as nonactive pregnant women

NOTE: A *trained* woman can tolerate 30 minutes of aerobic workout without increasing pulse greater than minimum.
Active women exercise at least 30 minutes 3x/week.

12

Exercise During Pregnancy

Pregnancy is quite a bit like a marathon. It is physically demanding, takes a long time to complete, and requires that you have a last burst of energy in reserve for getting over the finish line. Fortunately, you don't have to be in marathon form for pregnancy. But being in shape, having strength, stamina, and a feel for your body's responses to physical demands, can be a big advantage.

While whipping your body into shape before pregnancy is (merely!) challenging and demanding to *you*, when you exercise *during* pregnancy you must also consider how the growing fetus may be affected. Pregnancy is a unique physical condition that brings with it special demands, challenges, and potential individual problems, so it's difficult to set accurate exercise standards for active pregnant women.

Most authorities agree that exercise guidelines during pregnancy should be based on the physical changes taking place, and have established general guidelines for the pregnant woman based on those changes. But keep in mind that general recommendations may not be appropriate for you. A very fit pregnant athlete may tolerate a more strenuous program, whereas an overweight, out-of-shape woman may have to be much more cautious.

PREGNANCY CHANGES THAT AFFECT EXERCISE

During pregnancy, the amount of oxygen your body needs increases as your pregnancy progresses—up to as much as 16 to 32 percent just before delivery. That means you will end up needing almost a third more oxygen just to do the things you normally do—go to work, watch

TV, brush your teeth—because of the increased demands of the fetus, placenta, and uterus. Oxygen consumption also, of course, increases with exercise. Thus the most dramatic increases in oxygen consumption would occur during exercise late in pregnancy.

On the other hand, because all normal weight-bearing activities during pregnancy require this higher energy output, some improvement in fitness seems inevitable unless you cut back activity. In other words, you'll get fitter just by being pregnant. The ability to produce this increase in oxygen consumption seems within the reach of most women, suggesting that they should be able to handle most of the same tasks they did prior to pregnancy. However, working capacity is affected also by a variety of conditions, including body build, environmental factors, what the work is, training and adaptation, and psychic factors, including motivation.

Pregnancy also requires a 50 percent increase in the work of the heart (called "cardiac output"). This increase peaks at the seventh month of pregnancy, and then holds steady until delivery. During labor, the heart has to work harder, too. A woman who has maintained aerobic fitness prior to pregnancy comes into pregnancy with a greater capacity to meet the demands of carrying and delivering a baby.

In general, target heart rates of pregnant and postpartum women should be set approximately 20–35 percent lower than would be appropriate at normal times. Women's cardiovascular systems vary a great deal in their response to exercise during pregnancy, even more than in the nonpregnant state. When you exercise during pregnancy you should measure your heart rate (by taking your pulse) during the activities, and stay below a maximum of 140 beats per minute. Women who are anemic, very out-of-shape, or overweight should be particularly careful about pushing themselves too hard during a workout—their heart rates can quite quickly shoot up past the safe zone.

TEMPERATURE: A CRITICAL EXERCISE FACTOR

An elevated temperature during the first trimester of pregnancy seems to increase the risk of congenital abnormalities (teratogenesis). That's why an obstetrician is so concerned when a pregnant woman runs a fever. The critical "core" (deep body) temperature at which risk occurs is 38.5° Centigrade (102° Fahrenheit).

During exercise, your temperature also goes up. Although most of the extra heat your body produces is lost into the air around you, some cannot be dissipated fast enough. The result: increased body temperature. The longer and harder you exercise, the higher your core temperature is likely to go. If heat loss through the skin is reduced because it's hot or humid weather, your body is even less able to get rid of the excess.

The temperature of the fetus averages about half a degree Centigrade higher than that of the mother. Most of the heat the fetus produces is transferred to the mother across the placenta via the blood—much the way the body core is cooled by sending heat to the skin via the blood. (If the mother's temperature is elevated, the fetus cannot transfer its heat.) If the major determinant of fetal temperature, then, is the maternal body temperature, the temperature rise during exercise may become critical. Studies on this effect are the basis for the recommendations for exercise at the end of this chapter.

One study of five pregnant women doing *strenuous* exercise—such as exercising during hot weather or exercising vigorously in an aerobic dance class for an hour, followed by a session in a sauna or hot tub—revealed they had core temperatures of 0.3° to 0.5° Centigrade higher than had nonpregnant women. Strenuous exercise for 15 minutes, however, will not usually increase the temperature over 38° Centigrade. Pregnant women should, therefore, be cautioned not to exercise when they have a fever or too long in hot weather. And they should not add insult to possible injury by lingering in a hot tub or sauna after exercise.

HOW THE FETUS RESPONDS TO MATERNAL EXERCISE

The flow of blood to the uterus decreases the harder and longer you exercise. This would appear to mean there is a reduction in the supply of oxygen and nutrients to the fetus. However, this is not necessarily true, because the concentration of red blood cells in the blood increases during exercise, enabling the blood to carry more oxygen. The net result appears to be a fairly constant oxygen supply to the uterus and the fetus.

Fit people in general also have less of a reduction in blood flow to various organs during exercise, suggesting that the in-shape pregnant woman is better able to maintain blood flow to the uterus during exercise. How does the fetus respond to any changes in blood supply? Most studies show that the fetal heart rate rises *after* maternal exercise but it may actually *decrease* during exercise. However, there is a great deal of variation in answers from experiments designed to study the fetal heart rate's response to maternal exercise. Results differ with different stages of pregnancy, the intensity and duration of the exercise, even the position the exercise is done in. It is also difficult to monitor the fetal heart rate during exercise.

In general, however, it appears that upright, weight-bearing exercises (running, walking) cause greater changes in fetal heart rate (rising slightly) than non-weight-bearing swimming, rowing, or bicycling. However, no association has been found between such heart rate changes and subsequent problems in the newborn. And in no studies, even with moderately strenuous exercise, did the fetal heart rate show signs of stress. Stress changes would be very low or high rates or certain abnormal patterns.

Fetal health has been studied in relation to varying degrees of exercise. But it's very hard to pin down the effect of one single factor, such as exercise, because there are so many other variables—genetic, socioeconomic, nutritional, environmental, and stress-related. Also, the effects of strenuous exercise during pregnancy have been studied mainly in women who were already highly trained before pregnancy. All these studies show normal or improved fetal health, and while that might have been anticipated—these athletes began pregnancy in excellent condition and health—it does suggest that there are no major negative effects of strenuous exercise on the health of fetuses in *healthy* women.

The most commonly noted negative effect of strenuous exercise during pregnancy is low fetal birth weight. Some studies have reported a decrease of as much as 400 grams (one pound). However, this may reflect poor nutritional status of these women, or other factors than just the physical activity per se.

The effect of exercise may be positive or negative during pregnancy, depending on many factors. However, if you follow the guidelines on the following pages there should be no negative effects.

PSYCHOLOGICAL BENEFITS OF EXERCISE DURING PREGNANCY

In general, people who exercise report fewer feelings of anxiety and stress as well as a greater degree of self-confidence, self-control, and self-esteem, than those who are more sedentary. I believe that exercise may also help the pregnant woman feel physically and psychologically healthy, especially if she exercised routinely before pregnancy. Exercise may also help reduce the pregnant woman's anxiety about the birth process itself. A woman who feels strong and in control of her body before and throughout her prenatal period is more likely to feel secure during her labor and delivery.

EXERCISE SPECIFICS

The goal of exercise during pregnancy should be to maintain the highest level of fitness possible, with maximum safety in mind. That means you won't run faster or farther than ever before, or try for the same level of strength-training that would be reasonable if you weren't pregnant.

The following exercise program is designed for a broad spectrum of women. It incorporates modifications required by the physical changes of pregnancy and the postpartum period, and by a special concern for safety. Some women may be able to tolerate more strenuous exercise. Others may need to cut back even more, to, say, a simple walking program. There is enormous variability in the way different women will respond to the same activity, so no single exercise "prescription" can meet the needs of all women. Your obstetrician should assess your abilities and needs individually and help you construct a program that works for you.

The importance of this communication between you and your physician cannot be overemphasized. But you have to take responsibility, when you're out on the track or tennis court, for being alert to the potential hazards of exercise, aware of the warning signs, and for reporting back to your physician if anything unusual occurs.

Of course, your exercise program is only one part of a healthy pregnancy lifestyle. A daily walk won't cancel out a junk food diet, smoking, or not getting enough sleep. But taken with all the other healthy approaches to pregnancy, exercise can help you feel better, stronger, more energetic. And that can make a *big* difference.

The following guidelines are those outlined by the American College of Obstetricians and Gynecologists (ACOG) in their home exercise programs. (These programs are available on videotape; write to "Feeling Fine Programs, Inc.," 3575 Cahuenga Blvd., Los Angeles, Calif. 90068.) They are general, conservative criteria for safety and provide a good starting point.

ACOG EXERCISE GUIDELINES

The following guidelines are based on the unique physical and physiological conditions that exist during pregnancy and the postpartum period. They outline general criteria for safety to provide direction to patients in the development of home exercise programs.

PREGNANCY AND POSTPARTUM

1. Regular exercise (at least three times per week) is preferable to intermittent activity. Competitive activity should be discouraged.
2. Vigorous exercise should not be performed in hot, humid weather or when you have a fever.
3. Ballistic movements (jerky, bouncy motions) should be avoided. Exercise should be done on a wooden floor or a tightly carpeted surface to reduce shock and provide a sure footing.
4. Deep flexion or extension of joints should be avoided because of connective tissue laxity. Activities that require jumping, jarring motions or rapid changes in direction should be avoided because of joint instability.
5. Vigorous exercise should be preceded by a 5-minute period of muscle warm-up. This can be accomplished by slow walking or stationary cycling with low resistance.
6. Vigorous exercise should be followed by a period of gradually declining activity that includes gentle stationary stretching. Because connective tissue laxity increases the risk of joint injury, stretches should not be taken to the point of maximum resistance.
7. Heart rate should be measured at times of peak activity. Target heart rates and limits established in consultation with the physician should not be exceeded.
8. Care should be taken to gradually rise from the floor to avoid lightheadedness from falling blood pressure. Some form of activity involving the legs should be continued for a brief period.
9. Liquids should be taken liberally before and after exercise to prevent dehydration. If necessary, activity should be interrupted to replenish fluids.
10. Women who have led sedentary lifestyles should begin with phys-

ical activity of very low intensity and advance activity levels very gradually.

11. Activity should be stopped and the physician consulted if any unusual symptoms appear.

PREGNANCY ONLY

1. Maternal heart rate should not exceed 140 beats per minute.
2. Strenuous activities should not exceed 15 minutes in duration.
3. No exercise should be performed while lying on your back after the fourth month of gestation is completed.
4. Exercises that employ the Valsalva maneuver (strong bearing down) should be avoided.
5. Caloric intake should be adequate to meet the extra energy needs not only of pregnancy, but also of the exercise performed.
6. Maternal rectal temperature should not exceed 99.6° F.

SPECIAL EXERCISES FOR PREGNANCY AND THE POSTPARTUM PERIOD

☐ *Exercises for the back* are not recommended during pregnancy after the fourth month because they require a woman to lie on her back or bear down. The back is subjected to significant stress at this time and during the postpartum period, and many traditional back-strengthening exercises would add risk. As the fetus grows it puts pressure on the major vein carrying blood back to your heart (vena cava) on the right side of the abdomen. One exercise that can be done throughout pregnancy, however, is the "pelvic tilt," which strengthens abdominal musculature and reduces the lower lumbar lordosis. Pregnant women are encouraged to perform this exercise as many times as possible throughout the day.

☐ *Pelvic tilt.* Lie on the floor on your back with your hands at your sides and your knees bent. Slowly flatten the curve at the small of your back, pushing your spine down against the floor. This move is called a "pelvic tilt" because to do this, you are tightening your abdominal muscles (they should feel tight to the touch) to tilt, or rotate, your pelvis and eliminate the normal curve in the lower back. After holding the tilt position for a couple of seconds, relax your belly muscles and allow your spine to return to its relaxed position, curved up slightly off the floor. Repeat several times.

After delivery, back pain and injury remain a significant problem because of the repeated bending, lifting, and carrying associated with child-rearing. At this time, a full program of strengthening and stretching exercises for the abdomen, back, and legs can be incorporated into your daily program. The pelvic tilt should still be continued.

☐ *Exercises for the pelvic muscles (Kegel's exercises)* are simply the alternate tightening and relaxing of these muscles, an isometric technique. The physical and hormonal changes of pregnancy cause relaxation of the pelvic supporting tissues. Vaginal delivery stretches these tissues even further. Most women are not troubled by these changes, but some will complain of discomfort or of incontinence of urine. Others may be concerned about looseness of the vagina during intercourse.

Exercise will not alter major anatomic defects. However, in patients with mild pelvic relaxation, the regular use of Kegel's exercises may be all that is necessary to provide symptomatic relief in the postpartum period. Such patients should be taught how to perform these exercises and encouraged to use them. To get a feel for which muscles to squeeze, practice starting and stopping the flow of urine when you urinate.

WHEN NOT TO EXERCISE

RELATIVE CONTRAINDICATIONS

Your physician will need to evaluate each patient individually with respect to an exercise program. The following conditions may make vigorous physical activity during pregnancy undesirable:

- Hypertension
- Anemia or other blood disorders
- Thyroid disease
- Diabetes
- Cardiac arrythmia or palpitations
- History of precipitous (very fast) labor
- History of intrauterine growth retardation (cases where fetal and newborn size is smaller than average)

- History of bleeding during present pregnancy
- Breech presentation in the last trimester
- Excessive obesity
- Extreme underweight
- History of extremely sedentary lifestyle

ABSOLUTE CONTRAINDICATIONS

If you have any of the following conditions, you should not do *any* vigorous exercise during pregnancy:

- History of three or more spontaneous abortions
- Ruptured membranes
- Premature labor
- Diagnosed multiple gestation
- Incompetent cervix
- Bleeding or a diagnosis of placenta previa
- Diagnosed cardiac disease

You must be aware that complications arising during pregnancy that may make vigorous activity dangerous for a woman who was previously able to exercise without restriction.

In addition to these ACOG Guidelines, I want to enlarge on some special points that in my experience have proven important.

- Prepare for pregnancy by increasing your aerobic fitness and building your cardiac reserve even before you conceive. Having established a good workout exercise program beforehand, you will feel better and have an easier time continuing to exercise *during* pregnancy.
- Consult your physician at your first prenatal meeting and stress your exercise history, current exercise program, and what you would like to continue throughout pregnancy. Your exercise routine should be well within your physical limits: Do not push too hard.
- Consider decreasing weight-bearing aerobic exercises like aerobic dancing, rope-jumping, jogging, and running. Concentrate on bicycling, swimming, calisthenics, and stretching. These non-weight-bearing workouts cut down on bouncing, are a bit less strenuous,

and may be better tolerated by the fetus. Even if you are an avid runner, it's probably best to decrease the length and pace of your runs by your seventh month. This will probably feel natural to you, since this is when the fetus goes on a growing spree and your weight and balance will change quickly.

- Avoid risky activities such as mountain climbing, sky diving, motorcycle riding, strenuous horseback riding, gymnastics, and downhill skiing. As your pregnancy progresses, the increase in weight, the shift of your center of gravity, and the changes in your joints and ligaments will affect coordination and balance. Therefore, activities requiring very precise body control may be dangerous.
- Exercise regularly—at least three times a week, so long as you are healthy—to maintain your cardiac reserve and muscle tone. Sporadic exercise is much more stressful to your body.
- Exercise for shorter intervals, like 10 to 15 minutes; then rest for 5 minutes; then exercise for another 10 to 15 minutes.
- Decrease your exercise level as pregnancy progresses after seven months. Your increased body weight will demand a larger energy output, so you may feel more fatigued and reach your exercise limit sooner. A sensible rule of thumb is to forget everything about your old exercise regimen, how long, how fast, how intensely you worked out, except for how it *felt*. If you keep the *feeling* of exercise intensity steady, or even a bit lower, you'll naturally cut time, speed, duration, and the rest as your weight increases and other body changes occur. If you are a runner, decrease your mileage and speed drastically during the last four weeks prior to delivery.
- Take your pulse every so often while you are exercising. If it is more than 140 beats per minute slow down until it returns to 90, then build back up a bit. Your pregnancy maximum is 140.
- Avoid becoming overheated for extended periods. It is best not to exercise for longer than 35 minutes *total*, even less in hot, humid weather. Do not forget that, as your body temperature rises, so does that of your fetus. Limit the time spent in hot tubs, saunas, and baths: Stay in a sauna (below 178° Fahrenheit) for less than 5 minutes; stay in a hot bath (water below 102°) for less than 15 minutes.
- Avoid extreme stretching of joints because of the softening of connective tissue during pregnancy.
- Warm up and cool down. Five minutes of low-intensity exercise— walking, leisurely pool laps, easy biking—prepares the body grad-

ually for more strenuous exercise. This is important to prevent strain or injury. A 5-minute cool-down after exercise will let your breathing, heart, and metabolic rates ease back to normal gradually.

- Rest for 10 minutes after exercise by lying on your left side. This takes the pressure off the vena cava and promotes return circulation from your extremities and working muscles to your heart; this increases blood flow to your placenta and fetus. (Get up slowly to avoid dizziness or faintness after this or any other period of lying down.)
- Drink two or three large glasses of water after exercise to replace body fluids lost through perspiration. When exercising, stop to drink water every fifteen minutes. A few sips help even if you aren't thirsty, since thirst often lags behind your body's need for water.
- Increase your caloric intake to balance the calories burned during exercise, as stated before. Eat enough to achieve a weight gain of approximately one-half to one pound weekly beginning in your fourth month. Fish, low-fat cheese, eggs, and lean meat are your best add-ons.
- Wear a supportive bra and good sports shoes. Your increased breast size and overall weight gain mean you'll be much more comfortable—and safer—if you opt for good support gear.
- Stop exercising immediately if you have shortness of breath, excessively rapid heartbeat, dizziness, numbness, tingling, vaginal bleeding, passage of fluid from the vagina, or abdominal pain. Call your doctor to report the problem as soon as possible, and certainly before resuming exercising.

One last thought: By training and exercising during pregnancy, you may also be training your fetus for a better start in the marathon of life.

13

Environmental Hazards to Pregnancy: Drugs, Medications, and Chemicals

So-called environmental hazards to healthy pregnancy can crop up in what we normally think of as the environment—air, water, and soil—or from things like drugs and x-rays that become part of our "environment" when we get sick. Such hazards may arise from things you choose to do, such as smoke cigarettes, consume alcohol, drink coffee, or use various recreational drugs. They may also come from things we may not be aware of, or over which we have no direct control, such as toxic substances in food, water, or air, pesticides, food additives, industrial pollution, and contaminants.

It is important to realize that environmental hazards can affect reproduction not only by affecting pregnant women and their unborn offspring. The damage can be done long before a woman gets pregnant—damage to her eggs, for example. Environmental hazards can also affect men—leaving them sterile, or producing mutant sperm that are incapable of normal fertilization.

When exposure occurs during pregnancy the harmful effects are extremely varied, often depending on the stage of fetal development. Different kinds of damage may occur during the pre-implantation period, during the embryonic stage, during the third to the twelfth week, and during the fetal period (after 12 weeks of gestation). Sometimes there may be long-term disabilities in offspring that do not become apparent until childhood or even adulthood, such as development of behavioral disorders or cancer.

TOXINS AT WORK

The number of chemical and physical agents that pose a potential threat to some aspect of reproduction is enormous. Industries may be using more than 100,000 chemicals, of which only a small portion have been tested for their possible effects on men's and women's reproductive capacity or their direct impact on a developing fetus. While most chemicals have been tested for possible carcinogenesis (the ability to cause cancer), the standards for reproductive safety in occupational exposures lag far behind. The following is a table of some of the chemicals that are *known* to be hazardous to reproduction.

MEDICATIONS THAT ENDANGER PREGNANCY

Between 1957 and 1962 thousands of people took a drug called Thalidomide as a tranquilizer. Since it was available with or without a prescription, people assumed it was a safe drug. Inevitably, it was taken by some pregnant women—many of whom didn't even know they were pregnant at the time. The problem was that, taken between the twentieth and the twenty-fifth days after conception (only about two or three weeks after a missed period), Thalidomide interfered with the development of the fetal limbs. In the most severe cases, babies were born without arms and legs. Of course, as soon as the association was confirmed and publicized, Thalidomide was taken off the market. But not soon enough to undo the tragedies it had caused. As horrifying as this event was, it focused much-needed attention on the effects of drugs on pregnant women and their fetuses. It was a stimulus to intensify drug safety studies, and underscored the extreme caution that must be used in prescribing *any* drugs during pregnancy.

Another example of a long-term effect of a drug taken during pregnancy is the occurrence of vaginal cancer in the daughters of women who took diethylstilbestrol (DES) during pregnancy to prevent miscarriage. With DES there was an extra problem—detecting an association between a medication given to a mother before her child's birth that had an effect only after that child developed her own female organs. This link was made because one physician's suspicion was

TABLE 5

Hazardous Occupational & Environmental Exposures

EXPOSURE	POSSIBLE OUTCOME
Anaesthetic gases (operating room)	Spontaneous abortion Prematurity Fetal malformations
Lead (paint)	Spontaneous abortion Low birth weight Abnormal sperm production
Mercury (food contamination, certain industries)	Cerebral palsy Mental retardation
Beryllium and Selenium (jewelry industry)	Pregnancy precipitates increased level of disease in chronic beryllium poisoning. May cause teratogenesis (birth defects)
Polychlorinated biphenyls	Low birth weight Intrauterine growth retardation (IUGR)
Dioxin derivatives (herbicides)	May cause spontaneous abortions, IUGR
Pesticides	Decreased sperm production
Benzene solvents (dry cleaning & other industries)	Increased menstrual flow Anemia Bleeding disturbances
Carbon disulfide (textile industry)	Medical disorders of various types Decreased fertility Excessive fetal loss (miscarriage, stillbirth)
Chemicals at toxic waste dumps	Possible spontaneous abortions and IUGR

aroused when he discovered multiple cases of a type of cancer that should have been very rare. (For more on DES, and its effect on women who are now old enough to bear their own children, see Chapter 21, "Medical Problems in Pregnancy.")

A list of drugs now known to be dangerous during pregnancy includes: cancer-fighting drugs (such as alkylating agents and antimetabolites); some antibiotics (such as tetracycline—which can cause teeth to be stained and underdeveloped—and chloramphenicol); DES; hormones like estrogen, synthetic progesterone, testosterone; alcohol; cigarette smoke; narcotics; anticoagulants (such as Coumadin), Dilantin (an antiseizure drug), Thalidomide, Lithium (used to treat manic depression), Valium (a muscle relaxant and antianxiety drug), and tranquilizers (such as phenothiazines).

The list of possible hazardous drugs is long and varied. Your physician should be contacted before you take any medication while trying to conceive or while pregnant. One useful source book is *Handbook for Prescribing Medication During Pregnancy*, by R. Berkowitz, M.D., published by Little, Brown and Company, 1981.

ALCOHOL

It was only as recently as 1973 that a clearly defined group of newborns' problems due to alcohol was given the name "fetal alcohol syndrome." More than 50 percent of infants born to alcoholic women have features of the syndrome: growth retardation, brain and spinal cord abnormalities, and characteristic facial changes. Since the initial report of fetal alcohol syndrome (FAS), numerous cases have appeared in medical journals. Right now, however, the main concerns are: 1) what is the minimal dose of alcohol that will produce adverse effects; and 2) when, during pregnancy, is the fetus most vulnerable?

Severe fetal alcohol syndrome occurs only in children whose mothers were "heavy" drinkers during pregnancy. A decrease in alcohol consumption by heavy drinkers before pregnancy results in less growth retardation in infants than that observed in women who continued to drink heavily. However, adverse effects of alcohol, as measured by psychological testing, have been seen in infants whose mothers quit drinking early in pregnancy.

Some, but not all, studies have revealed significant drops in birth weight as alcohol consumption rises. Some studies have shown a greater frequency of malformations in children of alcohol users—even women who consumed less than two drinks a day or were "binge" drinkers (drank heavily only intermittently). Other studies have failed to confirm these latter findings. The stillbirth rate among women consuming at least three drinks a day was found to be two and a half times that of women drinking less than this amount. Spontaneous abortions are more than twice as common in pregnant women drinking moderately twice a week or more.

All this leaves the obstetrician, and women who are either pregnant or contemplating pregnancy, faced with a major dilemma of how much drinking—if any—is really safe. It might seem simple to just advise complete abstinence. But such a recommendation might not be followed, especially by the many women who have, in fact, consumed alcohol and produced absolutely normal and even exceptional children. Recommendation for abstinence might also cause considerable guilt and anxiety among women who drank before they knew they were pregnant. Finally, a total alcohol ban might even lead women to substitute other psychotropic (acting on the mind) drugs—which could be *more* risky—to relieve anxiety or fill the former role of alcohol.

In spite of its impracticality, the position that no risk of fetal damage will exist if the mother does not drink at all has been the official response. The Surgeon General's office has warned women to beware of not only alcoholic beverages but also small amounts of alcohol in some foods and drugs. Most other groups have taken a more moderate approach, advising of the hazards of excessive drinking and suggesting that this matter be discussed by each pregnant woman with her obstetrician. This seems the logical strategy until more information is available. It is the obstetrician, along with the patient, who must make appropriate decisions concerning alcohol consumption during pregnancy, as well as the use of other substances that put the fetus at risk. At the present time it is not possible to form rigid guidelines concerning a safe quantity of alcohol during pregnancy.

Caffeine

Caffeine has been shown to produce abnormalities in the offspring of laboratory animals. Surveys in humans have also suggested that excessive use may be bad for the fetus. In one study women consuming 600 milligrams or more of caffeine a day had a high incidence of miscarriage and prematurity. (Five ounces of coffee has approximately 100 milligrams of caffeine.) However, a more recent analysis of coffee consumption in 12,000 women did not reveal any relationship between prematurity or malformations and coffee consumption—once the impact of cigarette smoking was considered. I tell my patients attempting conception or already pregnant to cut coffee down to one cup per day, drink *weak* tea, cut out medications with caffeine (APCs, Empirin, Anacin, etc.), and watch out for excess cola consumption.

CIGARETTE SMOKING

Nicotine has been shown to restrict the blood flow through the placenta of laboratory animals. The carbon monoxide in the smoke is poisonous and the burning of the numerous toxic constituents of tobacco may contribute to this and other deleterious effects of smoking.

Smoking during pregnancy has been associated with lower birth weights, bleeding problems, more frequent miscarriages, stillbirths, and early infant deaths. Premature rupture of the amniotic sac increases in frequency in direct relationship to the number of cigarettes smoked.

Each cigarette cuts down the amount of nutrients and oxygen your fetus is receiving. My best advice is *don't* smoke at all; but if you must, use a low-tar brand, put it out after a few puffs, and cut down. Remember, your fetus is smoking with you!

OTHER DRUGS

The use of amphetamines during pregnancy has been linked to birth defects and low birth weight. Withdrawal symptoms have also been reported in infants whose mothers have used "speed." Cocaine has been shown to have similar effects; LSD has been associated with birth defects and chromosome changes. Marijuana causes birth defects in laboratory animals. Although its effect in humans has not been clearly defined, its use must be discouraged during pregnancy at this time.

In sum, adverse effects during pregnancy and the newborn period may be seen in varying degrees with almost all mood-altering drugs. It is obviously best to refrain from all such mood-altering substances during pregnancy. If it is not possible to completely eliminate substances such as caffeine and alcohol, due to ingrained habit, moderation is urged. If drug dependency has occurred, adequate therapy should be started. Gaining "independence" is tough, but well worth it for a healthy baby.

14

Genetic Counseling

Understanding of genetic disorders has increased dramatically in recent years as the science of medical genetics advances in giant steps. The new knowledge allows many couples to participate actively in their reproductive decision-making, where hopes and crossed fingers were once their only option.

As researchers uncovered the principles behind the inheritance of genetic abnormalities, they recognized that a small number of diseases followed specific patterns as they were passed from generation to generation, and that the likelihood of their occurrence in any particular couple could be known. Since then, there has been an astonishing increase in the amount of information gleaned from genes and even more so in the number of ways this information can be applied. For example, some genetic disorders that result in defects can be corrected *after* the baby is born. Some chromosome abnormalities and metabolic disorders can be accurately detected *in utero* with little risk to mother or fetus.

Couples come to genetic services by different routes. Some, especially those over thirty-five, simply come in, wanting to know what their genetic patterns reveal. Others have a relative who has been counseled; or a family physician, gynecologist, social worker, or clergyman has suggested the idea. Some couples have already given birth to a child with a genetic disorder or a congenital malformation and want to know the chances of the same thing happening again. Other people have bodies that bear physical signs of genetic problems or have a family member who does. A woman or her partner may be worried about the effects of exposure to known or suspected environmental hazards. And others may have a history of repeated miscarriages, or know they could be a carrier of a problem, and want to know if they have any detectable abnormal genes.

The number of individuals and couples seeking genetic services increases each year. The number of centers offering such counseling is also increasing. There are now more than 600 hospital-based genetic programs in the United States, with associated laboratory services to do studies. Some major medical centers have developed satellite clinics that reach out into surrounding communities to provide education and improved services. Your local medical school and the March of Dimes Program in New York City are good places to call for advice on finding a genetic counseling program.

The progress of medical genetics has come during a time when attitudes toward abortion and population control are evolving, but ethical, social, religious, and economic issues remain to be resolved. The choices a couple can be faced with are extremely difficult ones. They should not hesitate to lean on anyone available—especially each other—for emotional support. And they should dig up every scrap of information they can so that, whatever their decision, they feel it is right for them at that time and is based on medical knowledge and careful, honest self-questioning. Then a couple will know they've done the best they could under the circumstances.

BASIC GENETIC PRINCIPLES

Genetic disorders fall into three basic groups: chromosome, single gene or Mendelian, and multifactorial.

□ *Chromosome disorders* are "genetic," but they can be isolated accidents that are not passed from generation to generation. The cells of all living organisms contain a specific amount of genetic material in their nuclei, which generally stays the same throughout the organism's lifetime. This genetic material is arranged in distinct units called "chromosomes." Each chromosome is believed to contain hundreds, if not thousands, of genes; and each gene is responsible for a particular characteristic of the organism. In humans, every cell contains 46 chromosomes—in 23 pairs. Every cell, that is, *except* the reproductive cells, the ova of a woman and the sperm of a man. These come in "halves," each with 23 *unpaired* chromosomes, that will make a new, complete, unique combination of genes when they come together to form a new human being.

Of the 23 chromosome pairs in all nonreproductive cells, 22 pairs are called "autosomes." The last pair, the sex chromosomes—or X and Y chromosomes—determine whether the person is male or female. A normal human female is designated "46 XX" because she has the correct total chromosome number (46, or 23 pairs), one of which is XX and makes her female. A normal male is "46 XY"—he too has a total chromosome number of 46, that is, 22 autosomal pairs plus the single X and the single Y chromosome that make him a man (see Figures 16 and 17).

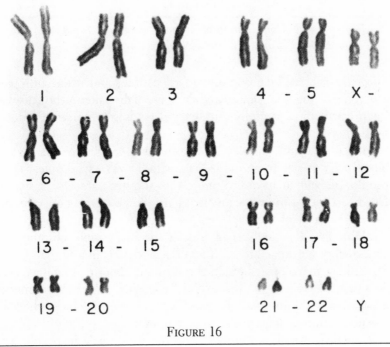

FIGURE 16

Illustration of 23 chromosome pairs. This pattern has two X chromosomes and is that of a female.

Chromosome analysis can be done on the white cells in the blood, cells in the bone marrow, skin cells, or the cells shed from a fetus into the amniotic fluid. The cells are grown in tissue culture so that some can be caught at the precise time in the division process when the individual chromosomes can be seen—in a normal, nondividing cell

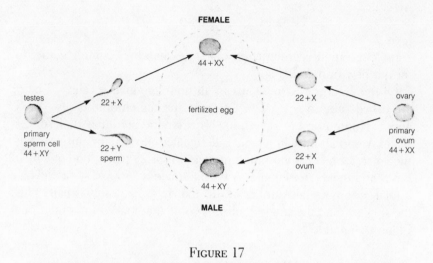

FEMALE

44 + XX

fertilized egg

testes

22 + X

22 + X

ovary

primary
sperm cell
44 + XY

22 + Y
sperm

22 + X
ovum

primary
ovum
44 + XX

44 + XY

MALE

FIGURE 17

Male or female: Combination of X and Y chromosomes made a male. Combination of X and X made a female.

they're invisible. The chromosomes are counted and arranged in pairs according to the size, shape, and dark-and-light patterns they display. Each pair is then carefully numbered according to a uniform identification system.

In 1959 an extra "number 21" chromosome was discovered in white blood cells grown from individuals with Down's syndrome. These people are said to have "trisomy-21"—another name for a type of Down's, which simply means they have "three number 21 chromosomes," instead of the expected two. This was an amazing genetic breakthrough: It was the first time a specific, visible chromosome abnormality was linked to specific physical defects in a human being. Since then, many other human chromosome abnormalities have been documented, some, like trisomy-21, associated with a structural alteration of the autosomal chromosomes' genetic material, others associated with a change in the sex chromosomes.

It's logical that these initial discoveries were made in people with obvious problems—abnormal sex characteristics, physical malformations, mental retardation, or diseases such as leukemia. But it was extremely surprising that, eventually, laboratory studies on cells from people who appeared absolutely normal sometimes had extreme chromosome deviations. Genetics is clearly an area in which much is left to be learned.

Chromosome disorders are classified as "genetic" because they involve genes. They are not necessarily "genetic" in the way most people think of the word: They can be one-time mutations that spontaneously occur at the time of early cell division, and are not inherited or passed on to offspring in succeeding generations. However, most chromosomal disorders *are* inherited.

Chromosomal surveys done on infants show that approximately one in 200 has a major chromosome variation, which may or may not have a negative impact on the baby's life. The most frequently seen chromosome disorder is trisomy-21, or Down's syndrome, which occurs in approximately one in 600 live births.

□ *Mendelian or single gene disorders*   occur when one member of a pair of genes is abnormal. More than 2,000 genetic variations of this type have been discovered by charting inheritance patterns, although how often most of them occur is unknown. These disorders follow the now-classic patterns first described by Gregor Mendel in 1865. Remember that genes containing specific biochemical information occur in pairs which are located at specific places in the chromosomes. Normal individuals receive one gene (half of each gene pair) from each of their parents. Mendelian "single gene" disorders are classified according to the way they are inherited—autosomal dominant, autosomal recessive, or X-linked recessive.

"Autosomal dominant" means the problem, whatever it is, will show up when just one abnormal gene is present. That single gene will "dominate" over the other normal one. These problems are thought to arise through spontaneous mutations, which can then be passed directly from one generation to the next. It is estimated that a person with a known autosomal dominant condition has a 50/50 chance of transmitting the mutant gene to his or her child. There are over 1,200 autosomal dominant disorders known today, and new ones are being uncovered all the time. Although these are generally not familiar names, one example is neurofibromatosis—the "Elephant Man's" disease. Of course, not only genetic *problems* are inherited in the autosomal dominant manner. Brown eyes are dominant over blue: one blue-eyed gene from Mom and one brown-eyed gene from Dad produces a brown-eyed kid.

"Autosomal recessive" conditions occur when both members of a particular gene pair are abnormal. A person is said to be a "carrier" if he or she has only *one* abnormal gene: The single gene isn't strong enough alone (as the "dominant" genes are) to make the carrier have a disorder; but he or she can pass it to children. If two carriers of the same abnormal gene have children, there is a 25 percent (one in four) chance that their offspring will receive a "double dose" of the harmful gene and actually have symptoms of the disorder. Statistically, a carrier couple like this has *the same* 25 percent chance with each pregnancy of giving birth to a child with a recessive disorder: The chances don't go up or down depending on whether one child does or doesn't have the disease. But the couple also has a 50 percent (two in four) chance of having a carrier child; and a 25 percent (one in four) chance of having a child with no abnormal genes at all. (Recessive genes also are involved in inheritance of normal traits. Remember, blue eyes are recessive. Only if two brown-eyed parents both have a gene for blue eyes does each child have a one in four chance of having blue eyes.)

There are over 900 known autosomal recessive disorders, including many disorders of metabolism, such as Tay-Sachs disease. Babies born with this disease (but *not* carriers) lack a specific enzyme which results in the buildup of a fatty substance in the cells of the brain and spinal cord. Symptoms—neurological problems—first appear in infants at about six months; death is inevitable by about four to six years. There is no treatment for this disorder. It occurs primarily in Jews of Eastern European origin, with a frequency of approximately one in 3,000 live births. Sensitive, reliable genetic tests can determine the carrier state in prospective parents, and amniocentesis can determine the genetic status of a fetus of carrier parents.

Phenylketonuria (PKU) is another metabolic problem passed by autosomal recessive inheritance. Here, too, an enzyme is lacking that is necessary for normal central nervous system function. In most states, inexpensive, simple, and accurate tests for PKU are the law for newborns. If affected babies are put on a special diet from birth, a substantial amount of otherwise inevitable mental retardation can be prevented. However, there is no carrier test available for PKU.

"X-linked recessive disorders" are problems that occur primarily in men but are passed along by women. This occurs because, as I've explained, men have one X and one Y sex-determining chromosome while women have two Xs. So if a woman inherits a single X gene for one of these diseases, she won't *have* the disease—since in recessive disorders the single healthy X will dominate—but she will be a carrier, capable of passing on that one abnormal X to a child. Men, on the other hand, have only a single X gene. So if they inherit a faulty X, they will have the disorder. There are approximately 150 X-linked recessive disorders, including hemophilia and Duchenne muscular dystrophy.

☐ *Multifactorial disorders*   are due to the interaction of many gene pairs with one another and with environmental factors (X-rays, drugs, etc.). Multifactorial disorders result in congenital malformations such as cleft palate, cleft lip, and defects of the nervous system. The frequency of these disorders is unknown, but the risk of recurrence in subsequent children is low.

GENETIC COUNSELING

Genetic counseling is a very detailed, complex, and time-consuming undertaking. The first thing the genetic counselor does is determine the reason a couple or person is seeking counseling. Then a complete history, or "pedigree," will be obtained. All past and present medical problems are reviewed, and information about age, nationality, habits, diet, hobbies, education, and vocation is included. Exposures to various infections and environmental hazards, such as x-rays and chemicals, are investigated. If a couple has had a child with a genetic problem, the counselor may review all information about its conception, other abortions or stillbirths, and the couple's methods of contraception. The counselor will study all available records, including birth, medical, and autopsy reports, and sometimes even family records and photographs if available. A physical examination will sometimes be done, and consultations with neurologists and ophthalmologists may be set up. Biochemical and chromosome tests may also be run.

All the data are then assembled and reviewed and a diagnosis is made. If there is a problem the counselor must first decide if it is genetic or environmental. If it is genetic the type of inheritance is figured out. The diagnosis and exactly what it means to a man, woman, or couple will then be explained in an interview. Mode of inheritance, recurrence risk, and, finally, all possible options are fully explained and considered, sometimes in writing as well as verbally.

CARRIERS OF GENETIC DISORDERS

The ability to detect carriers of genetic disorders can sometimes seem a double-edged sword. Screening programs, available to test populations at risk for such disorders as sickle cell anemia and Tay-Sachs disease, provide valuable genetic counseling, but are also responsible for suddenly changing couples who were previously unaware of their risk into couples with very real, very specific problems.

Genetic disorders—and carriers of them—are no longer viewed as a threat to society's well-being, but rather as an individual or family problem. Being labeled a carrier is an understandably upsetting experience—so much so, in fact, that some people may avoid genetic studies and all the benefits that can follow good counseling, because they fear they simply couldn't deal with the knowledge.

Carrier detection may have an enormous impact on mate selection and childbearing decisions. For example, those found before marriage to be carriers of a recessive disorder may, after counseling, decide to restrict their choices of mates in order to prevent the birth of abnormal children. Deciding when to tell this to a potential mate is an extremely difficult task; this is just one small example of the kind of pressure this knowledge can bring. Carrier detection after marriage brings its own set of problems, which may lead to discord and even divorce. Parents of a child with a genetic disorder are usually devastated, frightened, and full of grief and guilt. Studies of mothers of hemophiliac children suggest that their severe guilt may come from their perception of themselves as being genetically responsible for their baby's condition.

Much more needs to be learned about the effects of disclosing the carrier state, so that doctors, friends, potential and actual mates, and the carriers themselves can better cope with this extraordinarily difficult situation.

GENETIC PRENATAL TESTING

The use of amniocentesis and the new technique of chorion villous biopsy are prime examples of the way genetic advances in sterile laboratories can benefit actual women in real-life situations. These techniques (explained in detail in Chapter 20, "Prenatal Testing") remove fetal cells so their genetic makeup can be determined. Such prenatal diagnosis usually provides reassuring news. The vast majority of these studies show the fetus is normal. When these tests do reveal a genetic problem in a fetus, couples have the option of terminating the pregnancy.

Unfortunately, while prenatal testing can rule out a number of problems, it can't guarantee a healthy baby. Diagnosis is still not possible for many congenital abnormalities or Mendelian single gene disorders. For example, prenatal testing can determine the sex of a fetus in X-linked disorders such as hemophilia, but *not* whether the fetus actually has the disease.

All women should have knowledge about prenatal tests and the kinds of information they can and cannot provide. Current genetic counseling, fetal diagnosis, and screening for carriers of problematic genetic traits have all made great advances. Sometimes, however, to a couple caught in the middle of a terribly difficult situation, it may seem that what is known simply isn't enough. That is true, in many ways, and will continue to be true for the foreseeable future. But sometimes a little bit of knowledge can make a big difference. In many cases, genetic innovations have reduced human suffering. For information on genetic counseling contact your local medical center or the National Genetics Foundation, 555 West 57th Street, New York, N.Y. 10019.

15

The Prepregnancy Checklist

It still might seem a bit of an odd idea that pregnancy takes so much preparation, especially when millions of people have obviously gone through the process haphazardly, accidentally, with no planning *at all*, and have produced perfectly normal babies. But, of course, we aren't talking about just any pregnancy. We're talking about *your* pregnancy, whether it's planned for next month or the next decade. And you wouldn't be reading this book if you didn't already have the determination to "do pregnancy" with as high hopes and as rigorous demands for excellence as in everything else in your life.

I've gone over the basics of fitness, nutrition, and contraception, and tried to explain both how the healthy female body functions and how problems, when they do arise, can be taken care of so that they have the least possible impact on a woman's future fertility. I've outlined what women over thirty and working women can expect to be different about their pregnancies. I've sketched the basics of genetic counseling and provided an alert about the chemicals that can affect reproduction at work, at home, and in the environment. The checklist ahead is, in essence, a capsule summary of what has gone before. It's an at-a-glance reminder of all the things a health-conscious couple should take care of *before* they take the final step—conception. If you aren't sure exactly what's involved in one of the steps ahead, check back in the section about it earlier in the book.

BEFORE YOU CONCEIVE . . .

- Stop smoking. The ideal is to give your body a period of adjustment—say, six months. Short of that, throw away your last pack of cigarettes with your last packet of pills or when you tuck away your diaphragm or have your IUD removed.
- Cut down on alcohol. The official word from the Surgeon General is that no alcohol should be consumed during pregnancy. Since that period would include the critical time before you'll even know for sure that you are pregnant, the ideal would be no drinking from the time you start trying to conceive. If that seems unreasonable, ask your doctor to suggest more workable guidelines.
- Maximize nutrition. If you have weight to lose, try to drop it. A few pounds to gain, start eating! Remember these things take time—a two-pound weight change per week in either direction is a safe, healthy maximum. But that's not all: Even normal-weight women often have remarkably catch-as-catch-can eating habits. It's time to change this too. A body built on a strong nutritional bedrock is likely to have a healthier, easier time supporting pregnancy.
- Get fit. Pregnancy is a physical challenge. And like any other physical challenge, it will be accomplished most comfortably with a strong, fit body. Since it's not a good idea to tackle a get-in-shape plan once you are pregnant, the time for physical conditioning is before conception. You wouldn't run a marathon without months of training, and you shouldn't approach pregnancy as any less of a challenge.
- Dental checkup. Although almost any dental work can be done during pregnancy if necessary, why worry about the possibility? Also, your dentist may want to see you more frequently during pregnancy because of gum changes brought about by pregnancy hormones, so set up a schedule now.
- Gynecologic checkup. Three to four months before conception you should have:
  —a breast, pelvic, and general physical examination
  —a Pap smear
  —tests for sexually transmitted disease
  —blood tests as indicated, such as hemoglobin, blood sugar, and liver tests
  —a rubella test—and immunization, if necessary

—a toxoplasmosis (rare infection from raw meat, fish, and cats) test if you have or have had a cat
- Genetic screen. If there's any question of family diseases on either the man's or woman's side, check it out. Black couples should check for sickle cell trait. Jewish couples should test for Tay-Sachs carrier state.
- Avoid drugs, medications (unless approved by physician), x-rays, and environmental hazards while trying to conceive.
- Stop birth control. The Pill should be stopped three months before you try for a pregnancy. An IUD can be removed a month or two ahead of time. Barrier methods should be used during the intervening months, then stopped with your period when you want to start trying to conceive.

PART IV

Pregnancy

Introduction

It's finally time, you're ready for pregnancy! And after all the years you may have spent trying to *avoid* pregnancy before you were prepared to carry, deliver, and nurture a child, you may be surprised to discover that achieving pregnancy can take longer than you'd expect. I'll tell you why, and explain when and if something needs to be done about it. Now is also the time to learn about the changes you can anticipate in your body and your emotions in the months ahead, and about the importance of prenatal care—that close contact with the professional who will watch over you throughout your pregnancy, right up to the time your baby is delivered.

There are also subjects no one likes to think about at a time like this, but that are important to understand, just in case. A miscarriage or a tubal pregnancy will be much easier to deal with, both physically and emotionally, if you have an idea of what they're like, and how they affect your chances of having a healthy baby in the future. Also, if you have any special medical problems which could make for a high-risk pregnancy, like diabetes or high blood pressure or epilepsy, your primary physician may have you consult a specialist. This shouldn't be frightening. It should be taken as just one more sign that your doctor is doing everything possible to keep you healthy so your baby has a better chance of being healthy, too.

Depending on certain factors, your doctor may also recommend special tests during your pregnancy. You've probably heard the names before (amniocentesis, ultrasound, fetal monitoring, and more), and I'll tell you why each is done, what it feels like, and what it can reveal about the health of a developing fetus.

Pregnancy is truly one of the most extraordinary experiences of a woman's life. And, as with many things, the good parts can be even more exhilarating and the bad ones a little easier to cope with if you understand what's going on. It also helps to have an open and comfortable relationship with your obstetrician, so that anything you don't understand or are worried about can be put in perspective as quickly as possible.

16

Becoming Pregnant and Early Pregnancy

You have made the decision to have a child. And you have prepared for pregnancy by getting a thorough gynecologic history and physical examination, screening for conception, and counseling if necessary, plus eating, sleeping, and exercising in the healthiest possible way. Now, what do you actually need to know about becoming pregnant? Starting a much-wanted pregnancy isn't always as simple as you might think. But knowing a bit about the most common hurdles, as well as some of the complexities of the process of conception in the most straightforward of cases, can go a long way toward easing the stress of waiting for "the big event."

FERTILIZATION

Fertilization is defined as the moment when the male reproductive cell, namely the sperm, enters its female counterpart, the ovum, thus starting the process of pregnancy. From that second, this microscopic bundle of genetic material has all the basic elements it needs to develop from embryo to fetus and, finally, to newborn infant. As discussed in detail in the chapter on the menstrual cycle, the female ovary usually releases one egg each month into the reproductive tract to be fertilized. This process, called "ovulation," usually occurs ten to fourteen days before the next menstrual period starts, no matter how long a woman's cycle is. A woman with a twenty-eight-day menstrual cycle will, therefore, ovulate about two weeks after the onset of one period and two weeks before the next—right smack in the middle of the twenty-eight days. The woman with a thirty-day cycle, on the other hand, will still tend to ovulate about fourteen days *before* her next period, which means approximately sixteen days after the last cycle started. And a woman with a thirty-eight-day cycle will ovulate on day twenty-four, which is fourteen days before her next period starts. (Remember, a menstrual cycle is defined as beginning with the first day of bleeding and ends with the first day of the next period.) If you keep track of the length of your menstrual cycle over six months—marking each "day one" on your calendar, for example—you will start to get a fair idea of when you can expect ovulation (see Figure 8, p. 53).

Once the egg is released it is pulled into one of the Fallopian tubes by the fringelike fimbria at the tube's end. From there the egg is moved along by the tube's muscle squeezes and the brushings of tiny hairlike cilia that line it. It's in the tube that the egg meets the oncoming sperm, millions of sperm from a single ejaculation. Once fertilization happens, the egg takes about three days to travel down into the uterus. The uterine lining, or endometrium, has been built up during the cycle to receive and nourish the fertilized ovum. If the egg is not fertilized, it and the uterine lining will be discarded during the process of menstruation. Then the whole cycle begins again.

When the sperm are ejaculated at the top of the vagina during a woman's fertile period, the cervical mucus will allow the sperm to swim, lashing their tails, through the cervix, into the uterus, and out into the Fallopian tubes. Sperm can live about two days within the female reproductive tract. Intercourse, therefore, must occur within 48 hours of ovulation for conception to occur (see Figure 18).

With that in mind, you can start to formulate a plan for increasing the chances of fertilization each month. Once you have figured out about when ovulation will occur, and keeping in mind that sperm will live for forty-eight hours, you might want to try having intercourse at least three times around the projected time of ovulation. More specifically, in a twenty-eight-day cycle, ovulation is expected on about day fourteen. So if you have intercourse on days ten, twelve, fourteen, and sixteen, live sperm are most likely to be present at suitable intervals to achieve fertilization (see Figure 18). There are other methods of determining ovulation time, such as basal body temperature and chemical tests, mentioned elsewhere.

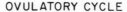

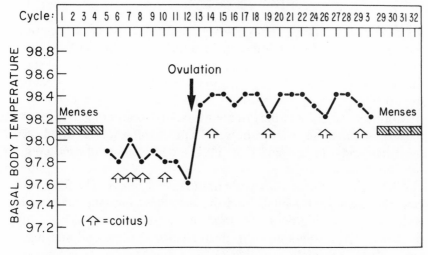

FIGURE 18

Timing of ovulation with sexual intercourse. Intercourse should occur prior to rise or on rise of basal body temperature to achieve a pregnancy.

EARLY PREGNANCY

"Implantation" is the name of the process by which the fertilized egg burrows into the lining of the uterus. The process starts two to three days after the fertilized egg reaches the uterus, and may be marked by a small amount of vaginal bleeding, which can last a few days. Once implantation occurs, the endometrium nourishes the fertilized egg and allows it to develop.

If an embryo *does* implant into the lining of the uterus, menstruation does not, of course, occur. During days twenty-one to twenty-eight of the menstrual cycle, before a period would even be late, there is rapid growth of the fertilized egg and the placenta begins to develop. The placenta is the embryo's life-support system, providing food and oxygen to the fetus and whisking away urine and carbon dioxide, the waste products of fetal metabolism.

By the end of what is called the first month of pregnancy the fertilized egg is actually about fourteen days old and is smaller than a pea. The placenta has begun to produce a hormone called "human chorionic gonadotropin" (HCG). This is the main hormone of pregnancy and is the stimulus for many of the changes in the mother's body during the course of her pregnancy. The first traces of this hormone can be detected in the mother's blood by very sensitive tests called "immunoassays," as early as nine days after fertilization. The level of this hormone then rises rapidly as pregnancy continues. (HCG is also the substance that home pregnancy tests detect. More on them coming up.)

Around six weeks after the last menstrual period the embryo is about the size of a marble. In the four weeks since fertilization occurred, its heart has begun to beat and there is early development of ears, eyes, nose, and brain.

After eight weeks the fetus is about the size of an egg. The fetus has external organs and genitals, and the protective amniotic sac, filled with shock-absorbing fluid, surrounds it. An ultrasound "picture" of the fetus at eight weeks shows its heart beating. (Ultrasound imaging, also called "sonography," is done by bouncing harmless sound waves through the mother's abdomen, and translating the result into a picture of the inside of the uterus.) By this time mild intrauterine cramps may be felt by the mother. These twinges, which may feel like mild menstrual cramps, are perfectly normal as long as they are not accompanied by vaginal bleeding.

By twelve weeks the fetus is the size of a tennis ball, and has developed tiny fingers and toes, complete with nails. Four weeks later, at four months, the fetus is about seven inches long and weighs less than half a pound. Sonography at this time may reveal "breathing" and "swallowing" movements and it's often not long—usually sometime during the sixteenth to twentieth weeks—before the mother first feels the movements of the fetus's arms and legs as it "swims" in its pool of amniotic fluid, an event called "quickening." Although these movements may be so subtle at first that they may even resemble mild intestinal movements, as they become stronger there's no mistaking what they are. By this time your physician can usually hear the tiny fetal heart with a stethoscope, thumping steadily at a quick 140 beats per minute.

PREGNANCY TESTING

The measurement of human chorionic gonadotropin (HCG), the hormone produced by the placenta, is the basis of all current pregnancy tests. This hormone was first detected in the urine of pregnant women in 1927, by two researchers named Ascheim and Zondeck. At first, HCG could be measured only indirectly—in laboratory animals, rab-

TABLE 6

CHRONOLOGICAL LANDMARKS OF EARLY PREGNANCY

WEEKS 1–4
Day 1:	Last menstrual period
14:	Ovulation or fertilization
14–20:	Migration of fertilized egg to uterine cavity
20–23:	Implantation
23:	Positive blood test for HCG hormone
21–28:	Rapid growth of fertilized egg
	Development of early placenta
	Pregnancy 14 days old; smaller than pea
29–33:	Development of positive home pregnancy test

WEEKS 6–8   Pregnancy size of marble
Circulation system develops

WEEK 8   Heartbeat "seen" on ultrasound
Pregnancy size of hen's egg

WEEK 9   Chorionic villous biopsy test can be done

WEEK 12   Pregnancy size of tennis ball
Fingers, toes, & nails develop (a miniature human being)

WEEK 16   Fetus seven inches long
Breathing & swallowing reflexes developed
Amniotic fluid increases—amniocentesis can be performed
Alpha-fetoprotein test done

WEEKS 16–20   "Quickening" can be felt
Fetus ten inches long
Uterus at navel

bits for one example. (This is where the term "rabbit test" came from.) The animals were injected with a woman's urine and examined after a period of time for ovarian changes that would indicate that HCG was present. The process took days and was not completely reliable.

Very recently, pregnancy testing methods have been developed that are done directly on a woman's blood or urine and that produce very rapid and reliable results. A kind of test called "radioimmunoassay" (RIA) is so sensitive it can detect HCG in the blood just nine days after conception and only one day after implantation. But since RIA blood tests are expensive and a blood sample must be drawn by needle, they are not used routinely. Urine tests, on the other hand, make getting a sample to test easy. However, conventional urine test methods, the home version or the laboratory type, were only sensitive enough to become positive after the twenty-sixth day of conception or thirty-eight to forty days after the last menstrual period.

Very recently urine testing has achieved a breakthrough that puts it close behind blood testing in speed and accuracy, while maintaining the advantage of easy sampling—that special boon that makes urine testing a way every woman can have access to pregnancy diagnosis in her own home. The difference is "monoclonal antibodies"—the result of state-of-the-art technology—that are designed to react *only* with HCG, making the test extremely accurate. (Earlier tests also tended to react with a hormone called "LH," produced in a woman's body after ovulation. It was possible, then, for old tests to read positive when a woman wasn't pregnant if the test was done just after ovulation.) This new kind of pregnancy test kit has just recently come on the market—"e. p. t. plus" is one brand to look for. Other advantages of this new breed of home tests are that movement or vibration, which could obscure results in the older type of kits, does not affect an accurate reading at all. You can even carry the kit with you until it's time to check it. At the end of two hours: a color change means pregnancy; no change means no pregnancy. And, finally, you can get these quick, precise results just nine days after a missed period.

Pregnancy testing—early, accurate pregnancy testing—is more than just a way to satisfy a woman's very understandable curiosity about whether or not she is pregnant. The sooner she knows, the sooner she can be even more careful of her good habits—eating healthily, getting enough sleep and regular, moderate exercise—and cut out possibly harmful ones—smoking, drinking, and drug taking. Home tests can offer an additional bonus: They allow a couple trying for pregnancy the privacy to savor the excitement of a positive result together, if only for a few hours or days before going to the doctor. And a negative result can save couples from the time and expense of an unnecessary doctor visit.

Besides just using HCG to confirm a pregnancy (a kind of "yes/no" evaluation), measuring the precise amount of HCG in the blood has become an important tool in the hands of your physician, as well. Having several checks of the HCG levels (called a "BSU pregnancy blood test") over a period of time can shed valuable clues as to whether or not a pregnancy is healthy. For example, an impending miscarriage can sometimes be predicted by the fact that BSU levels fail to rise. Ectopic pregnancies (those that implant out of the uterus, most often in the Fallopian tubes) can be diagnosed by low levels of BSU. Many physicians obtain a "baseline level" of BSU when a woman has had a previous abnormal pregnancy or if there is any suspicion that the current one may present problems.

Becoming Pregnant Can Take Time

It may surprise many young couples, especially those who have been careful and diligent about birth control for many years, that pregnancy doesn't always happen as soon as they decide to try for it. In fact, it will take that average couple about four to six months to achieve a pregnancy. After a year of trying, 80 percent of couples will produce a pregnancy. If conception does not occur after one year of intercourse without birth control, it's time to seek expert advice. When the woman is over thirty or the man is over fifty, a medical evaluation is in order after six months of trying. It is expected that these couples may take longer to achieve pregnancy. But, at the same time, they have fewer fertile years left in which to evaluate and treat any problems that may be present. (Difficulty conceiving is discussed in detail in Chapter 22, "The Causes of Infertility.")

But no matter what your age, it's best to just relax and have fun with sex during the time you're trying to get pregnant. Try not to keep deadlines at the back of your mind or adhere to schedules of "prime times" for conception. Taken to extremes, the stress of trying to get pregnant can even throw off your menstrual cycle—just as any stress can—and make pregnancy even less likely. This is a unique time for most people. There are no worries about remembering pills or pauses to insert a diaphragm or put on a condom. That freedom, and the excitement of what's ahead, can make this a time of very special pleasure.

17

Prenatal Care: Healthy Pregnancy "Insurance"

Modern care of a woman during pregnancy has made both gestation and childbirth safer than many of the other challenges we face in modern life. To make sure the process proceeds as smoothly as possible, it is important for every woman to visit a physician as soon as she thinks she is pregnant. Suspicions confirmed, it's time to begin prenatal care, the special form of health care that helps ensure the delivery of a healthy baby by a happy mother.

During pregnancy the fetus doesn't really reveal that much about its condition in the safe, cushioned environment of the womb. Your physician will want to see you on a regular basis, to look for any signs and symptoms that could indicate trouble. The absolute ideal in prenatal care, as I have said before (and will say again!), really begins *before* pregnancy. By the time most pregnancies are confirmed, six or more weeks following the last menstrual period, most of the fetal organs have already formed. The circulatory system and major sense organs are well developed. To make those first critical weeks count for mother and child, preconception care should have included complete medical, dental, and gynecologic examinations, plus all the other healthy lifestyle changes I've discussed.

DUE DATES: "WHEN WILL THE BABY BE BORN?"

As soon as a woman knows she's pregnant, she quite naturally wants to know, "When will my baby be born?" This can be estimated by a simple formula. Note that I say "estimated"—"guesstimated" might be more like it! "Due date" only represents an average time. Don't plan on delivering *on* that date—or you will most likely be disappointed. Plan for *around* that date.

Since the exact time of ovulation or conception cannot be precisely pinned down, we calculate the due date from something that can be: the first day of your last menstrual period. A simple formula based on the average length of pregnancy—which is 266 days, or 38 weeks—will give an estimated date of delivery. Take the first day of your last menstrual period, add seven days, and count back three months. So, if your last period was March 1, add seven days (March 8), then count back three months to December 8, and you will have your estimated delivery date.

However, only one baby in ten arrives on the exact due date. Those aren't great odds! There is less than a 50/50 chance that labor will start within a week of the estimated date. The length of pregnancy varies greatly in the same woman as well as from woman to woman. And, obviously, women with irregular menstrual cycles have even less chance of "guesstimating" the correct due date.

We don't stay totally in the dark for the whole pregnancy, however. Due date uncertainties can be offset by our ability to track the growth of the uterus and the fetus. Serial BSU blood tests (explained further in Chapter 16, "Becoming Pregnant and Early Pregnancy") and ultrasound examinations (see Chapter 20, "Prenatal Testing") have also tremendously improved the accuracy of estimating the due date. You yourself can make a rough estimate when you detect some movement of the fetus. Many obstetricians believe in ultrasound screening of every woman during the first five or six months of pregnancy. This will accurately determine the dates of pregnancy.

Toward the end of pregnancy another symptom, called "lightening," occurs. This means that the baby's head drops into the cradle of the pelvic bones in preparation for birth. This generally happens two weeks before delivery, but (no surprise) it can take place earlier or later.

Many couples decide to keep the due date to themselves so that they will not start pinning too many hopes on a particular day. Excited, well-meaning friends and relatives can inadvertently add to the anxiety,

asking, "Haven't you gone to the hospital yet?", "Aren't you overdue—
is everything all right?", and similar questions. Pregnancies *can* be
prolonged, a situation we call the "postmaturity syndrome." Babies
that are more than two to three weeks post-term do have an increased
risk of problems. However, this is uncommon—it occurs only in about
4 percent of all pregnancies.

The other side of the coin is the "premature" baby. Prematurity is
defined not by age, but as a birth weight under five and a half pounds.
Twins average earlier deliveries by about three weeks, about the 245th
day of pregnancy.

Many of the feelings of anticipation during a pregnancy are due to
the fact that the baby keeps its parents guessing about its exact time
of arrival. Get used to it.

CHOOSING YOUR DOCTOR

There are several options for medical care during your pregnancy.
Your family doctor may care for you; or you may go to one of the
many fine available hospital clinics. Most couples, however, choose
a physician who specializes in obstetrics, that branch of medicine
concerned with pregnancy and birth. An obstetrician/gynecologist is
a physician who is totally devoted to preconceptional care, the management of pregnancy, labor and delivery, and postpartum care.

In England, "midwifery" carries the same meaning that "obstetrics"
does in the United States. In the United States there has been a
resurgence in the use of nurses trained as midwives who work directly
with physicians to deliver babies. This medical team may work in a
family health, or birthing, center, which is another alternative to the
private obstetrician. And, if money is a major concern, this last option
will probably cost less.

Today there is only one maternal death in 10,000 births; the vast
majority of those are of women who entered their pregnancies with
some kind of health problem. Before 1930 there was an average of 60
maternal deaths for every 10,000 live births. This dramatic reduction
is a testament to the increased quality of medical care. Many factors
are responsible for this reduction, including the development of antibiotics, transfusions, surgery, and—probably the most important factor—the extraordinary advancements in the field of obstetrics.

The American Board of Obstetrics and Gynecology, which certifies
specialists in the field, has very high standards. Doctors seeking cer-

tification must be graduates of accredited medical schools and must thereafter complete a four-year residency in an accredited hospital. After that they must practice in the specialty for several years, and *then* pass both written and oral examinations.

If there is no one who can recommend an acceptable physician to you, contact your local medical society and ask who, among its members, are board-certified obstetricians. Or you can write to the American College of Obstetrics and Gynecology in Washington, D.C., for a list of members in your immediate area.

In recent years a superspecialist in obstetrics, called a "perinatologist," has evolved, who has spent additional years in training for the care of problem pregnancies. This expert is usually associated with a major medical center and offers consultation in cases of high-risk pregnancies.

If you are interested in care by a midwife, I would recommend a hospital-based midwifery practice with backup by a physician. The American College of Nurse Midwives (1522 K Street N.W., Washington, D.C. 20001) may also be of help.

YOUR FIRST VISIT

You will probably be anxious on your first visit to the doctor for the confirmation of your suspicion that you are pregnant. You may have already performed a home pregnancy test, such as e. p. t. plus. These over-the-counter test kits are very reliable if performed carefully, and can be done as early as a few days after a missed period. Your physician, by examining you, and by doing either a blood or urine pregnancy test, can confirm your home diagnosis. You will want the doctor to give you some instructions to follow during this very special period of early pregnancy.

Your past obstetrical history, which includes a brief account of each former pregnancy, delivery, miscarriage, or abortion, will be taken. You will be asked about any medical problems you may have had, previous infections, or venereal diseases, and any family history of genetic problems.

On completion of the history a complete physical examination will be performed and your blood pressure measured. Blood pressure is an important number to note, because if you should show an abnormal rise in blood pressure late in pregnancy, it may indicate the development of toxemia, a serious condition which occurs only in pregnancy. You will be weighed, and the result will become a reference point for how much you gain and how quickly you do it.

Blood samples will also be drawn. The level of hemoglobin, the oxygen-carrying protein of red blood cells, will be measured. Too few red cells indicate anemia, which is very common among pregnant women. If you are anemic during pregnancy you will probably tire more easily and your body will not be able to support your own health and the growth of the fetus as well as it might otherwise. Fortunately, this condition is easily corrected with daily supplements of iron. Many doctors routinely prescribe iron as well as a special prenatal vitamin supplement.

In addition, the blood sample will also reveal your blood type, especially your "Rh" status. Rh-negative women married to Rh-positive husbands require special care during pregnancy (discussed at length in Chapter 19, "Problems of Early Pregnancy"). Other routine blood tests include those for syphilis, toxoplasmosis, rubella antibodies, and the presence of abnormal blood antibodies. Your physician will also check your urine for both protein and sugar. He or she will probably repeat this urine test on each visit thereafter to rule out the presence of diabetes or kidney abnormalities. Part of every visit, too, is an examination of your breasts.

A pelvic examination will probably also be performed, which will reveal a great deal of information. By feeling the uterus and measuring its size a pregnancy can be confirmed. The cervix and the lower uterus also become softer with pregnancy. Uterine enlargement can be felt as early as six to eight weeks after conception. The pregnant uterus can be felt through the abdomen after the third month of pregnancy. Between eight and twelve weeks, the physician may also be able to hear the fetal heart with an ultrasound transducer stethoscope.

A Pap smear will be done to rule out cervical cancer. The pelvic bones may also be measured to see if the birth channel is large enough to allow the passage of a term fetus.

Upon completion of the physical, your physician will outline the course of pregnancy and ask you to return every three to four weeks until the eighth month, when you will probably visit the doctor every two weeks. In the ninth month you will go every week, and sometimes more often.

On most of these routine visits your blood pressure, weight, and urine samples will be analyzed. Fetal growth will be measured by feeling the abdomen. Occasionally a vaginal examination will be done to more closely measure fetal growth, position, and size as well as to check the condition of the cervix. Many physicians do routine vaginal examinations during the ninth month to determine if the fetus's head has dropped into the pelvic bones, and to determine the condition of the cervix, to predict when labor might begin. Sometimes this examination is followed by very slight vaginal bleeding, but this is no cause for worry. Vaginal examinations by your physician are safe unless the amniotic sac is ruptured, when there would be a risk of introducing infection.

Instructions to pregnant women vary from doctor to doctor. But basically diet, exercise, bowel function, bathing, and general health are reviewed. The major goal of this examination is to check the health of the mother in early pregnancy and to start a plan for good obstetrical care. Warning symptoms may also be outlined by your physician. The general "do's-and-don'ts" of pregnancy will be discussed. Do not be afraid to ask questions. The more you know the less frightened you will be of the many changes your body will undergo and the more you will enjoy your pregnancy.

COMMON DANGER SIGNALS IN PREGNANCY

- Vaginal Bleeding. Twenty percent of all women report some vaginal bleeding during the first three months of pregnancy. Most of the time it is insignificant. However, since it may also be a sign of impending miscarriage, it is always important to consult your physician if you bleed.
- Severe Continuous Headaches. Headaches are common in pregnancy, especially in the first trimester. They may result from rhinitis, a sinus condition often occurring during pregnancy, or from the excess fluid retained by the body at this time. But headaches can also mean toxemia is developing, so they should be reported to your physician.
- Swelling of the Face and Fingers. This may be a simple sign of fluid retention or it may be another early sign of toxemia. Report it to your doctor immediately.
- Blurred Vision. It is common to require a change in contact lenses because of swelling of the cornea of the eye. Blurred vision is still another sign of fluid retention or of toxemia. Call your doctor.
- Severe Abdominal Pain. Intermittent contractions, known as Braxton-Hicks contractions, are normal. The abdomen may also be a

little sore from the rapid growth of the fetus. But constant or debilitating pain is not normal and should not go unexamined.

- Fever. This usually indicates your system is reacting to a virus or bacterial infection. However, a high temperature, even from a simple cold, can trigger premature labor. Fever should be reported immediately to your physician.
- Persistent Vomiting. Nausea and vomiting occur to some extent in 50 percent of all pregnancies and, by themselves, should be no cause for alarm. Persistent vomiting (more than two times a day) should be reported to your physician, however, because of the risk of dehydration.
- Vaginal Discharge. During pregnancy vaginal discharge usually increases, becoming thick and sticky. But a large amount of clear fluid discharge is not normal. It may be just secretion from the cervix; but it could indicate a leakage of the amniotic sac, the protective fluid "cushion" surrounding the fetus. Your physician should decide; let him or her know.

IMMUNIZATIONS DURING PREGNANCY

The following table summarizes the recommendations of the American College of Obstetricians and Gynecologists regarding the safety of various immunizations during pregnancy.

TABLE 7

IMMUNIZATIONS DURING PREGNANCY

Tetanus-diphtheria	Give if no previous vaccination or no booster in last 10 years
Polio	Not recommended routinely for adults
Mumps	Not safe during pregnancy
Rubella	Not safe during pregnancy
Typhoid	Recommended if traveling to high-risk regions
Smallpox	No need; disease has been eradicated
Yellow fever	Immunize only before travel in high-risk areas
Cholera	Immunize only before travel in high-risk areas
Hepatitis A	Immunize after exposure or before travel in developing countries
Rabies	Recommendations do not change for pregnancy
Influenza	Not safe for pregnant women with certain medical problems such as diabetes, severe anemia, and heart disease

18

A Time of Change:
Physical and Emotional
Reactions to Pregnancy

During the course of your pregnancy you will experience numerous changes in your body and emotions. Some (like swollen breasts, mood swings) you've probably anticipated; others (a stuffy nose) may take you by surprise. The symptoms of pregnancy vary greatly from individual to individual. Some women experience few or none at all; but if you do experience a couple you are certainly not alone. Almost all of these changes disappear after delivery. The most serious signs of problems have already been outlined. Refer to them often. But even some "normal" changes can be disconcerting, especially in first pregnancies. Of course, if any concern or frighten you, talk to your doctor. Don't worry about "bothering" your physician with "little" worries: He or she is there to evaluate any changes—that's part of the job—and make you as confident, relaxed, and comfortable as possible. That's good for you, *and* good for your baby.

COMMON SYMPTOMS DURING PREGNANCY

☐ *Braxton-Hicks contractions* (periodic uterine contractions that may start as early as the first trimester) begin as a tightening feeling at the top of the uterus, gradually spread downward, and then disappear. The contractions are exercising and strengthening your uterus for the hard work of labor ahead. In the late third trimester these contractions increase and may be responsible for early thinning (effacement) and opening (dilatation) of the cervix before labor actually begins.

☐ *Breasts may swell, tingle, and throb* during pregnancy as milk glands develop. The veins often become more visible because of increased blood supply to the breasts. The areola, which is the area around the nipples, and the nipples themselves may darken. Lumpy breasts are also quite common in pregnancy. However, if the breasts feel suspicious in any way—if lumps are hard or fixed or cause dimpling—discuss this with your physician.

Wear a support bra right from the start: Most of the weight gain in the breasts comes during the first half of pregnancy. If your breasts get very large it may be a good idea to wear a bra even at night. Lack of support during pregnancy may exacerbate sagging afterward. Hereditary factors also play a part in how much loss of tone you can expect in the breasts.

☐ *Nipple secretions* may occur during pregnancy. This sticky, yellowish, watery fluid is called colostrum, and will be the baby's first food. In the later months of pregnancy drops may form spontaneously on the nipples and may be expressed (or squeezed) from the nipples intentionally.

☐ *Muscle cramps* are common during pregnancy and may be due to changes in the blood supply to various muscles or to changes in calcium metabolism. (Calcium is involved in muscle contraction.) Shooting pains down your legs can be due to pressure of the fetus's head on certain nerves. Elevating your legs, and heating pads, may help ease cramps.

☐ *Dizziness or faintness* during pregnancy can be due to: 1) the enlarged uterus pressing on the major blood vessels and causing a blood pressure drop; 2) hormonal changes that cause a relaxation or widening of blood vessels so that blood pools in the legs. Move slowly to avoid sudden blood pressure changes, and assume new positions (especially from lying down to standing) gradually.

☐ *Gas,* or flatulence, is a common complaint of pregnancy. The stomach and intestines may swell and give you a bloated feeling. Laxatives may help, as will avoiding gas-producing foods like beans, cabbage, onions, and fried foods. Regular bowel movements reduce gas.

☐ *Hemorrhoids* are a well-known result of increased pressure on the veins in your anus. They are the lower bowel's equivalent of varicose veins of the legs. Avoiding constipation and straining when moving the bowels help to prevent hemorrhoids. Cold compresses with witch hazel are comforting to hemorrhoids that do form. Hemorrhoids generally become worse just after delivery and then gradually recede in the postpartum period.

☐ *Shortness of breath* sometimes occurs during pregnancy. Pregnant women take in more air for various hormonal reasons. Also, by late pregnancy the fetus is so large it borrows some of the space lungs normally expand into. This shortness of breath is nothing to worry about and is not a sign of heart and lung disease.

☐ *Backache* is one of the most common minor problems of pregnant women. It is caused by the changes in posture required by the growing, thriving fetus. Backache is usually best treated with heating pads, analgesics (check with your doctor first), a pillow to support the small of the back when sitting, a maternity girdle, and a firm mattress.

There are special exercises that may also help alleviate backache by strengthening the back muscles and relieving excess tension. Consult your physician, however, before starting any exercise program. Severe backache may be incapacitating and should be treated.

☐ *Constipation* is very common during pregnancy. Pregnancy hormones produce relaxation of the bowel, and decreased physical activity and pressure on the lower bowel by the growing fetus all increase the tendency toward irregularity. Most women who had very regular bowel habits before pregnancy can cope with the tendency toward constipation by drinking plenty of fluids, taking gentle exercise like walking, and using mild laxatives such as milk of magnesia, prune juice, and fibery whole-grain cereals. Avoid the routine use of harsh laxatives and enemas, because they may become habit-forming. Here, again, your physician is your best guide to the use of *any* medication, even those available without a prescription.

☐ *Excessive urination.* Having to urinate more frequently may become a problem as the fetus grows and presses on the bladder. "Every five minutes—even during the night!" I've been told more than once in mock seriousness. In the absence of burning or a constant urge to urinate, this is normal. The above symptoms, which suggest a bladder infection, should be checked out by your doctor.

☐ *Swollen ankles and varicose veins* develop in many women as the fetus grows and puts pressure on the veins in the legs. An inherited tendency may aggravate this condition, in which varicose veins are distended and swollen and may be painful and tender. They are aggravated by long periods of standing and by large weight gains. Many women find elastic support hose provide the best relief from discomfort. Support stockings vary in strength from mildly elastic "light support" to surgical stockings that are expensive and require expert fitting. Ask your doctor for suggestions.

☐ *Fatigue* tires pregnant women easily, especially in the first and third trimesters. A nap during the afternoon or going to bed earlier may help. If you are a working woman, try to rest during lunch and breaks.

☐ *Headaches* of mild intensity and duration are a common complaint, especially during early pregnancy. Although we do not know the cause, most disappear by mid-pregnancy. Simple analgesics, such as Tylenol, are helpful. Check with your physician to see what he or she prescribes, and to be sure your headaches are not severe enough to suggest other problems.

☐ *Heartburn* in pregnancy is due to the growing fetus pressing on the stomach, causing the mother's food to occasionally be pushed up into the esophagus, the tube that runs from mouth to stomach. Heartburn, actually irritation of the esophagus, causes a burning sensation in the lower chest or mid-abdominal region. The treatment consists of taking antacid medication and eating bland foods like bread, pasta, and milk. Sleeping on two or three pillows may also help by enlisting gravity to help keep food down where it belongs.

☐ *Nausea and vomiting* are among the most common problems of the first trimester of pregnancy: About 50 percent of women have them to some degree. Nausea may actually be your first clue to pregnancy—it can appear as early as the second week—but usually develops about the fifth week, or following a missed period. Symptoms may continue into the third month or longer. Most, but not all, women reported feeling sick after getting up or after breakfast—hence the moniker "morning sickness."

The cause of this nausea is not really known, although hormonal effects on the gastrointestinal tract are probably to blame. The treatment is quite simple: Most women find that frequent small snacks of dry foods (like graham crackers), small sips of liquids, and starchy foods (like rice and pasta) are helpful. Keep a couple of crackers at your bedside and eat them when you wake up. If vomiting is so persistent you can hardly keep anything down, let your doctor know.

☐ *Rhinitis: The pregnant nose* is what many women who develop it call postnasal drip, or a persistent feeling of nasal stuffiness caused by a swelling of the mucous membranes of the nose and throat. The "pregnancy rhinitis" is due to the effects of estrogen on these tissues. If it is annoying, appropriate medication can be prescribed by your physician.

☐ *Tooth decay* is not due to the old theory that the mother's teeth decalcify to provide calcium and phosphorus for the fetus. That is now known not to be valid. But while there is no evidence of an adverse effect of pregnancy on healthy *teeth*, chronic inflammation of the gums is common. This inflammation, due to the increase in estrogen, which boosts the blood supply to and thickens the gums, usually gets worse as pregnancy progresses. Routine dental visits should be scheduled during the course of pregnancy, and any cavities filled. Local anaesthetics for the treatment of dental caries will not harm the fetus in any way.

SKIN CHANGES DURING PREGNANCY

Although it may seem totally unrelated to what's happening inside your body, the skin is affected in many ways as a result of pregnancy.

Among early changes in the skin is a darkening of the nipple area. Women who have any warts, moles, or scars may notice them darken as pregnancy progresses. There is also a line from the navel to the pubic bone which may become very dark and then gradually fade out at the edges. This "linea nigra" is much more visible on more darkly pigmented skin. These areas fade following delivery.

Another condition, referred to as the "mask of pregnancy" or "chloasma," may vary from small, yellow-brown spots to extensive dark-brown patches on the nose, cheeks, and neck. Although sometimes unsightly, these patches are no cause for worry, since they disappear within a few weeks after delivery. (Some birth control pills, which mimic pregnancy hormonally, may cause the same skin discoloration.) A sunscreen may decrease the pigmentation, which tends to increase in ultraviolet light.

Sometime during the second trimester a woman may notice red spots on her face, neck, chest, and arms—"spidery"-looking because they have a tiny red center and threadlike branching "legs." These become more apparent as pregnancy progresses but disappear after delivery. A variation on these "spider spots" may appear on the feet, palms, and hands, causing them to become red and mottled. These skin changes are probably a result of the hormonal changes of pregnancy.

Some women find themselves sweating more heavily during pregnancy, especially after the third month. To avoid annoying skin conditions, such as heat rash, try to stay cool and dry; a light dusting of talcum can be used, and clothes should be loose and comfortable.

"Stretch marks" or "striae" are common during pregnancy, probably also due to hormone changes. These occur mostly on the swelling belly, but some may also appear on the breasts and thighs. On white skin these start as thin pink lines but may become dense and white and brown, and appear as loosely wrinkled skin. Striae are less common in black women. After delivery the pink color fades but narrow ribbons of silver-white remain.

During the second half of pregnancy there may be a gradual increase in the sensitivity of your skin to ultraviolet light. Be careful not to sunburn. Following pregnancy there may be some temporary hair loss, another condition attributed to withdrawal of the pregnancy hormones that have controlled hair growth for the past nine months. Be reassured that hair that thinned during and after pregnancy will eventually return to normal.

SURGERY DURING PREGNANCY

Facing surgery during pregnancy is a relatively rare problem. However, should the occasion arise it is reassuring to know that with an operation such as an appendectomy the woman and fetus are not usually harmed. In fact, delaying surgery in such emergency conditions is probably worse for the pregnancy.

The most common situations requiring surgery during pregnancy are appendicitis, trauma to the limbs (like broken bones), ovarian cyst operations, suspicious breast masses, and dental surgery. The doctor will distinguish between emergency surgery (which *must* be done at once) and elective surgery (which can wait, if necessary, until after delivery). My own advice is to postpone any elective surgery.

Anaesthetic techniques have now advanced to the point where, if surgery is required, safety precautions can be undertaken. Enough oxygen will be administered along with the anaesthetic so that mother and fetus will have plenty for both. Both mother and fetus can, if necessary, tolerate various anaesthetics without difficulty. Even specialized, extreme operations, such as open heart surgery, may be safely performed during pregnancy if necessary. Treatment for the incompetent cervix syndrome (discussed in Chapter 21, "Medical Problems in Pregnancy") is a common obstetrical situation requiring minor surgery during pregnancy.

EMOTIONAL REACTIONS DURING PREGNANCY

Most women realize that, in addition to physical changes, pregnancy can cause profound emotional reactions. Some of these are conscious feelings, such as the deep pleasure that comes from the confirmation of pregnancy; others are unconscious, such as the fear of bodily pain, or death. When a woman realizes that she is pregnant, even if the pregnancy is much wanted and carefully planned, anxiety and ambivalence coexist. Pregnancy, delivery, and the postpartum period may be marked by physical strain and psychological stress. Fear and uncertainty are frequently experienced in the same way as they are in any other major life change.

Extreme anxiety can interfere with labor and delivery and with being a parent, stemming from several different sources:

- worry about the effects of the baby on your relationship with your husband
- worry about not having the capacity to love and care for an infant
- a special deep preference regarding the baby's sex
- dread of having an abnormal baby
- ambivalence about giving up one's personal freedom.

It is important to recognize that some anxiety and ambivalence are absolutely normal. They do not mean you can't be a good parent, or that you weren't ready for pregnancy. Contrary to common sense, and probably against all evidence from friends and family who have been there themselves, many people persist in expecting pregnancy to be an idyllic time. It won't be. Pregnancy is, quite simply, too momentous an occasion to be contained by one small part of your emotions. One patient told me, "I'm a successful banker, two hundred people work for me, and I rise to every business challenge. But I'm scared stiff of having this baby." Another patient, a successful model, was vomiting a lot during pregnancy—it turned out she was scared of having an "ugly" child. A good doctor-patient relationship will make it possible for you to voice your fears: It is important to get your doubts out in the open (where a looming anxiety often shrinks to a more appropriate size) without feeling criticized or guilty.

Certain physical discomforts of the first trimester—nausea, vomiting, fatigue, and headaches—may bring a sense of disappointment that the expected feelings of excitement are not present. Moodiness is common. However, the second trimester is usually characterized by a sense of well-being. The unpleasant symptoms of the first trimester often disappear, and the excitement of feeling your baby move and seeing your belly swell contribute to this good feeling.

Often during the third trimester some discomfort and fatigue occur. There is also increased anxiety as well as insomnia. These *normal* fears center on the realities of being a mother, the inevitable changes in the marriage, concerns about labor and delivery, especially if there have been problems in the past, concern about the sex and health of the baby, and concerns about death or injury to yourself and/or the child.

EMOTIONAL ASPECTS OF HIGH-RISK PREGNANCY

A pregnancy following a period of infertility, the birth of an abnormal child, spontaneous abortion, or the loss of a child may be accompanied by understandably heightened anxiety. If a miscarriage has occurred in the past, a woman may wonder if she can carry the current fetus to term. She may fear that she has physical problems or is somehow a damaged woman. Listening to the fetal heart tones, seeing the fetus on ultrasound, and becoming involved with the progress of the pregnancy may all help to ease anxiety.

Pregnancy is generally a normal event. However, with the high-risk obstetrical patient, pregnancy is not normal. Living with the fear of losing an unborn baby is highly stressful. Feeling of guilt and blame are common. Worries about hurting the fetus during sex may create tension with your partner. Talk to your doctor about these feelings. If they seem out of proportion or otherwise too difficult to handle, your doctor may suggest seeing someone specially trained to help couples through this very difficult situation. One of my patients who had had three spontaneous abortions was overcome by terrible anxiety. Her problem was handled by scheduling an appointment every week so that she could listen to the fetal heartbeat.

SEX DURING PREGNANCY

There are marked individual differences in the effect of pregnancy on sexuality. Many women report increased desire, although pregnancy has also been reported to dampen sexuality. As a general rule, sexual interest and frequency of intercourse are reported to be higher during the first trimester than before pregnancy; above normal, but below the first trimester, during the second trimester; and decreased in the third trimester and after delivery. Fatigue, physical discomfort, and fear of harming the fetus are common interferences at the end of pregnancy.

Women may become anxious about their attractiveness before and after delivery. Many feel there's something not quite right about even showing their sexuality during pregnancy. Women who are pregnant— and facing the challenge of nurturing for the first time in their lives— may also experience an increased need for nurturing and physical contact themselves. If you are surprised by a disruption in your sex life and wonder whether this reaction is normal, a discussion with your obstetrician will help put things into perspective.

Fears About Labor and Delivery

No one doubts that women experience pain during childbirth. However, preparation, understanding, and a positive attitude can reduce that suffering. Consider the difference between repairing a two-inch cut on the arm of a twenty-two-year-old frontline soldier and repairing the same size wound on a confused and frightened three-year-old child. An adequately prepared woman may be as calm as the soldier; while a woman who does not understand what is going on might panic like the child.

For some women, delivery may be their first experience in a hospital. An earlier tour of the maternal area may help reduce fears associated with a hospital. Virtually all so-called psycho-prophylactic techniques (Lamaze is the well-known one) contain elements of education, physical therapy, and psychotherapy and, in many women, reduce the need for pain relief and anaesthesia. Women in such classes are educated in the anatomy and physiology of childbirth, trained to relax mentally and physically, and taught to concentrate on breathing exercises which distract them from the pain.

Many studies on the psychological factors relating to childbirth agree that the underlying factor in a positive childbirth experience is a woman's desire to be an active participant in labor and delivery. Prepared childbirth not only reduces pain, but it enhances the experience of birth and facilitates the bond between mother and child. Prepared childbirth has been shown to result in the use of fewer drugs and in higher levels of enjoyment of the process of childbirth.

But there are limits to what prepared childbirth can accomplish. If women set very rigid standards or have unrealistic expectations about delivery, these could cause difficulty when things do not follow a precise, predetermined course. If ideal labor is painless and the use of drugs represents failure, then a woman may feel that she did not "measure up" to natural childbirth if she didn't revel in every non-medicated contraction. Women should be prepared for the potential need for medical intervention, and the need for drugs. Understanding the use of medications ahead of time will avoid needless anxiety and help prevent women from feeling inadequate and guilty if they need them.

A difficult delivery can be traumatic and emotionally exhausting and may contribute to postpartum depression. Since women do most of the work involved in labor, even the most competent require support, encouragement, praise. That is where a husband—or friend or family member—plays a critical role.

Fetal monitoring can both ease and create anxiety. Monitoring, although a major advance in obstetrical care, may present a dilemma: It transforms the labor room into an intensive-care setting at a time when couples are seeking a more personal childbirth experience. Many women find the monitor a reassurance of the baby's condition during labor, but others find it an uncomfortable annoyance which interferes with labor, detracts attention from them, and provokes anxiety. Women should be fully advised when it is needed, be familiar with the equipment beforehand, and have their views about it considered. Women who have had problems with labor and delivery in the past—with previous obstetrical losses—more readily accept fetal monitoring and respond more positively to it. Fetal monitoring, when used sensitively and intelligently, can be an asset in the management of childbirth.

Family-centered obstetric care includes the father in delivery. This treats childbearing as a normal and healthy process—a major family experience. Fathers are now present in the labor and delivery rooms, even in the cesarean section room, much more often. They have become actively involved in the delivery process even to the extent of assisting in the delivery in some centers. A father's participation during labor and delivery provides emotional support to the mother, even during cesarean section. Some obstetricians may wish the father to leave should certain problems arise at delivery. In any event, the doctor's and hospital's policy should be discussed with the couple in advance.

Home births may seem to be gaining in popularity, but their number has actually remained constant at about 1 percent since 1977. A major deterrent is the fact that a complicated labor can follow a perfectly normal, uneventful pregnancy. Twenty percent of normal pregnancies may be followed by labor complications. The solution, therefore, would seem to be to make the hospital more homelike rather than take delivery back to the home. Caring, warmth, and attention on the part of the medical staff will help this occur.

BREASTFEEDING

The advantages of breastfeeding are now well documented. Breast-feeding is a normal biological function providing many recognized advantages to mother and infant. It may be started immediately after birth, in the delivery room. Breastfeeding promotes the normal transition beween symbiotic involvement of the pregnant woman with her fetus to the warm, nurturing relationship between mother and infant.

Many women report a sense of closeness with the infant, feelings of increased self-esteem, and sensual gratification from breastfeeding. Since some fathers feel shut out from this special relationship, they will feel less deprived if they are encouraged to feed the infant supplemental bottles and assist in the care of the newborn.

A complete discussion of breastfeeding is beyond the scope of this book. For further information consult *The Womanly Art of Breast-feeding*, La Leche League, and *Understanding Pregnancy and Child-birth*, S. H. Cherry, M.D., Bantam paperback.

19

Problems of Early Pregnancy: Miscarriage and Ectopic Pregnancy

The vast majority of pregnancies proceed normally. However, the purpose of prenatal care is to watch out for certain conditions of pregnancy which no one likes to talk about but which it is crucial to be aware of. Knowing what they and their danger signs are will help you to understand the nature of pregnancy and what can be done to ensure the best health for mother and child.

MISCARRIAGE

During the early part of pregnancy, most commonly during the first three months, there is a possibility of losing the pregnancy. This is called a "miscarriage" or "spontaneous abortion." If a pregnancy is not progressing normally, for reasons which we shall discuss, the lining of the uterus may begin to shed and bleeding may occur. Eventually the pregnancy separates from the uterine lining and passes out of the body. A naturally occurring miscarriage (spontaneous abortion) should not be confused with a planned therapeutic abortion, which is a voluntary procedure to end a pregnancy.

Medically, miscarriage is defined as the premature delivery of a nonviable fetus (one that could not live) before it weighs about one pound. This generally can occur up to about twenty weeks of pregnancy. However, over 90 percent of miscarriages occur within the first three months. Amazingly, the incidence of miscarriage may be as high as *half of all conceptions*. However, most of these early miscarriages occur before women even know they were pregnant. A very heavy, maybe slightly late, "menstrual period" associated with severe cramps may actually be a very early miscarriage. Studies have been done (on women who were trying to conceive) by doing pregnancy tests every month— *before* a missed period. Results revealed that many pregnancies aborted very early and without the women's knowledge. Of the pregnancies documented after a missed period, the incidence of miscarriage is approximately 15 percent. In women over forty the miscarriage rate may be as high as 30 percent.

A miscarriage is always a traumatic event in any family and may be followed by depression in both partners. Postmiscarriage depression is discussed on page 195. Spontaneous miscarriage, however, is most often followed by another pregnancy which results in the birth of a healthy baby. The vast majority of the causes of miscarriage will not occur again.

Usually two signals indicate that something is wrong and there is a chance of miscarriage: One is vaginal bleeding without the passage of tissue; the other is cramping pain in the lower abdomen. The cramps may come and go and are felt right above the pubic bone. Sometimes vaginal bleeding stops and pregnancy goes on without any problem whatsoever. At other times the bleeding and cramping may continue, becoming increasingly stronger until miscarriage occurs. In some ways a miscarriage is a less intense version of labor. The pain is usually stronger than menstrual cramps. If the bleeding is heavier than a menstrual period, and the cramps worse, that is not a good sign.

At the beginning of pregnancy, a few women may have slight bleeding when the fertilized egg attaches itself to the lining of the uterus. Some women may confuse this implantation bleeding with a normal, but light, menstrual period. A pregnancy test, however, will show early pregnancy.

Any bleeding during pregnancy should be reported to your doctor. Twenty-five percent of all pregnant women experience bleeding or spotting during the first three months of pregnancy. Only slightly more than half of these end up having a miscarriage. The others go on to deliver healthy babies.

If bleeding stops and the pregnancy goes to term, the baby is as likely as any other baby to be completely normal. This is a very important point, to reassure the many couples who fear—unnecessarily—that bleeding in pregnancy means that something is wrong with the baby.

☐ *The causes of miscarriage* are largely random and hard to foresee. In spite of all the wonders of modern medicine, doctors have absolutely no control over the vast majority of these causes. Not all the seeds you plant in your garden grow; not every fertilized egg can result in a normal baby. There may be something wrong with the sperm cell or the egg cell, or something may happen when they are joined that keeps the fertilized egg from growing properly.

Chromosome and Structural Abnormalities. A large number of miscarriages are caused by a spontaneous defect arising in a growing embryo during its early stages of development. Since most of the fetus is formed in the first three months, any serious problem will manifest itself by that time and the body will reject those fetuses that have problems. In one analysis of 1,000 miscarriages (the ejected tissues were studied), it was found that over half were caused by what is called a "blighted ovum." In these cases the embryo stops growing and dries up, and the amniotic sac ends up empty. There was something intrinsically wrong with that fertilized egg that did not allow it to develop.

Often there may be a month between the time the embryo stops growing and the actual miscarriage. The extreme is a "missed abortion"—when the body holds on to the dead embryo for two months or more. Once the fetus has failed to develop normally it is only a matter of time until the miscarriage occurs.

The causes of these abnormalities, which are forty times more frequent in spontaneously aborting fetuses than in normal full-term babies, are not known. They are just random accidents of nature. Given the many millions of sperm produced, and the thousands of ova, it is not really surprising that this can happen.

There are several factors that influence the frequency of spontaneous abortion. One is maternal age. The miscarriage rate doubles from an average of 15 percent in women ages twenty-five to forty to over 30 percent after age forty.

Other Causes of Miscarriage. There are certain maternal conditions that can result in miscarriage: abnormalities of the uterus (double uterus, septate uterus, uterine fibroids); an incompetent cervix (see p. 194); hormonal dysfunction (such as an "inadequate luteal phase," related to a deficiency of progesterone); thyroid dysfunction; and other hormonal imbalances.

Some infections—herpes, toxoplasmosis, rubella, cytomegalovirus, chlamydia, and mycoplasma—have been implicated in causing miscarriage. Severe acute infections associated with high fever, such as pneumonia and typhoid fever, sometimes can lead to spontaneous abortion.

Teratogens (substances such as radiation and certain drugs and chemicals that cause fetal malformations) can increase the miscarriage rate.

Pregnant women commonly fall or trip, probably because of a change in their gait or balance. In general, the fetus is well protected from these bumps. The uterus acts as a fluid-filled buffer if the woman is jostled during pregnancy. It is unusual for trauma of this nature to cause any problems. Remember that most miscarriages are due to random factors which will not occur again. Rarely does trauma result in damage to a pregnancy. Physical and mental stress are also usually not causes for abortion.

Genetic Causes. Couples who have had three or more miscarriages need genetic studies. Although rare, an abnormality of the chromosomes in one of the partners may allow pregnancy to begin but end in recurrent miscarriages.

□ *The course of miscarriage*   depends on whether or not the pregnancy is viable. A miscarriage is called a "complete abortion" if all the fetal tissue is passed spontaneously and none remains in the uterus. This is usually associated with severe laborlike pain of increasing severity, followed by the expulsion of a complete fetus and other pregnancy tissues. Bleeding and pain subside once the tissue is out, and the uterus reverts to normal size. Your physician will usually have you in for several checks without requiring any further procedures.

An incomplete miscarriage, which is more common, occurs when some fetal tissue remains in the uterus. With this type of miscarriage, vaginal bleeding continues from the tissue that remains. That tissue, if left in the uterus, may be the trigger for severe infection. For this reason, a dilatation and curettage (D&C), or opening of the cervix and scraping of the uterus, is required to remove the left-behind tissue. This can be done either in the doctor's office or in a hospital, with either regional or local anaesthesia. Women with Rh-negative blood must also receive a shot of Rh immunoglobulin after a miscarriage.

A missed abortion occurs when an embryo dies but is not expelled from the uterus. Diagnosis is made by ultrasound studies and blood tests that measure pregnancy hormone levels. A D&C will be performed in order to avoid the heavy bleeding which might have occurred when the body finally expelled the no longer viable pregnancy.

A threatened abortion is a situation in which bleeding occurs with some mild cramps but the pregnancy is still viable. Bleeding itself does not mean a definite miscarriage. However, the bleeding plus cramping is a more ominous sign. The treatment of threatened miscarriage is very individual and depends on the woman and her physician. The classic approach is bed rest and restriction of physical activity and sex. Some physicians use vitamins, hormones, and sedatives. Ultrasound and pregnancy hormone levels may differentiate threatened abortion with a healthy fetus from an inevitable abortion with a fetus that would not survive.

The use of ultrasound after vaginal bleeding has proven to be of great value. As early as seven to eight weeks after a last menstrual period, a fetal heart can be seen. If the fetal heart is beating healthily it is much more likely that a miscarriage will not occur. However, if a woman has bleeding after eight or nine weeks of pregnancy and ultrasound shows no fetal heart, then miscarriage is inevitable and a D&C can be performed.

Keeping track of blood hormone levels is of value in the early stages of pregnancy before the fetal heart can be detected. A healthy, viable pregnancy will have increasing levels of these pregnancy hormones during the first four months of pregnancy. This test is called a "quantitative beta sub unit HCG pregnancy test." Normally, the level of hormone doubles every two to three days.

Late miscarriages, occurring after ten to twelve weeks of pregnancy, are much less common, especially if the fetal heart has been heard and a missed abortion is ruled out. One cause of late abortion is a condition called "cervical incompetence": the cervix cannot hold itself closed once the fetus grows to a certain size in the uterus; the cervix slowly opens, eventually resulting in the loss of the pregnancy. The causes of cervical incompetence include previous surgery to the cervix, malformations of the uterus, and exposure of the mother to the drug DES when she was in her own mother's uterus. Sometimes no cause is discernible.

Treatment of cervical incompetence is very simple once the diagnosis is established. The doctor simply sews a stitch around the outside of the cervix, draws it tight, and knots it. This "purse-string suture" is left in place until the end of pregnancy, when it is removed to allow the birth of the baby. This procedure can be repeated with each pregnancy after twelve to fourteen weeks and once a viable fetus has been established.

☐ *Treatment of multiple miscarriages.* Since most miscarriages are due to random factors that will not usually repeat themselves, a work-up for miscarriage is usually not necessary until a woman has had three successive miscarriages without a live birth—or after two successive miscarriages if she is over thirty. Of course, this is a general rule; each case needs to be individualized, depending on many different factors. For example, late miscarriages following fetal viability should be evaluated.

A work-up for "habitual" abortion or miscarriage will include an x-ray of the reproductive system called a "hysterogram," which will reveal abnormalities or growths in the uterus. Hormone studies, including thyroid function tests, are also performed. Genetic abnormalities and infections in the couple need to be ruled out. Cultures for infections such as chlamydia and mycoplasm can be done.

Women who have had miscarriages, with or without a D&C, should wait two menstrual cycles before trying again for pregnancy. This allows the lining of the uterus to heal enough to be fully ready to receive and nurture the next pregnancy.

☐ *The emotional impact of miscarriage* is often so shattering that many couples blame themselves, despite the fact that spontaneous abortion is a natural event and the overwhelming majority of them are due to an intrinsic abnormality of the egg or sperm. In the great majority of cases the embryo was simply unable to survive. Like any accident, a miscarriage is regrettable, upsetting, but unavoidable.

The experience may have been frightening for you and your partner, and mutual support and compassion are very important. "It was terrible when I started to bleed in the restaurant. I was terrified all the way to the emergency room, and neither my husband nor I knew what was happening to me," said a young woman of her miscarriage.

Following a miscarriage a period of grieving is normal; you and your partner may feel a sense of loss and emptiness. Our society has no accepted ritual to support you during this kind of crisis. Talking with friends, physicians, and other people who have had a similar experience may provide comfort. "I didn't understand how I could be so wiped out by losing a baby I never even felt move inside me. But other

women—some of them friends I never knew *had* miscarriages—
told me they had felt that way too. That helped John and me tremendously," a woman who is now the mother of a healthy newborn
told me.

Most couples review their lifestyle to see if something they did caused
the event. Some even interpret a miscarriage religiously, as divine
punishment. This is guilt. It is unhealthy and unnecessary. Healthy
pregnancies remain intact even after strenuous activity and severe emotional disturbances—even after women *try* to induce miscarriages by
various (and *dangerous*) means. It is simply not the pregnant woman's
fault if she miscarries. Most important of all, try to look to the future:
This pregnancy loss will, very likely, be followed by a successful birth.

ECTOPIC PREGNANCY

Ectopic pregnancy occurs when the fertilized egg implants and grows
outside of the uterus. Most often (95 percent of the time, in fact) this
occurs in the Fallopian tubes, although ovarian or abdominal pregnancies are not unheard of. Misplaced pregnancies appear to be on
the rise: Now one in 100 pregnancies is ectopic.

Tubal ectopics occur when there is some kind of erratic trip-up in
the passage of the fertilized egg through the Fallopian tube. Blockage
in the tube may be due to scars left from an infection, endometriosis,
tubal surgery, pregnancy with an IUD in place, or a tubal abnormality
with which the woman was born. If the fertilized egg is delayed, it
may simply implant where it's stuck, since the environment in the
tube will allow implantation and development, at least for a short time.
The uterus, however, is the only organ that can accommodate healthy
implantation and full growth of a fetus. A growing ectopic pregnancy
will eventually burst the tube and often cause severe hemorrhage. A
woman can die if an ectopic pregnancy is not diagnosed and treatment
is delayed.

☐ *Symptoms of ectopic pregnancy.* During the first few weeks an
ectopic pregnancy usually appears perfectly normal. As the pregnancy
progresses, however, aches or twinges of pain may occur on the side
of the ectopic pregnancy. Vaginal bleeding may start, due to the insufficient hormone production of this abnormal pregnancy.

If you experience pronounced pain on one side of the lower abdomen, associated with a missed period or slight vaginal bleeding,

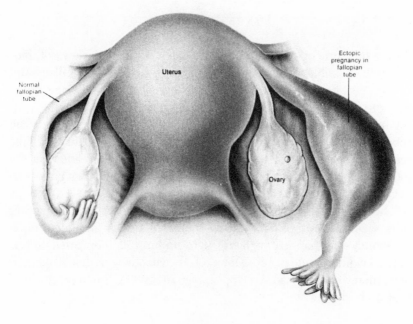

FIGURE 19

An unruptured ectopic pregnancy
Courtesy of Syntex Laboratories, Inc.

consult a doctor right away. The seriousness of ectopic pregnancy requires the physician to consider its possibility, do a pregnancy test and an ultrasound examination, and follow you very closely. Women who are at increased risk for ectopic pregnancies—who have had a previous ectopic, tubal surgery, or pelvic infection—should be followed even more closely.

The development of sensitive measurements of pregnancy hormones and ultrasound allows the diagnosis of ectopic pregnancy much earlier than, say, ten years ago. In addition, laparoscopy, which lets the physician actually see into the abdomen to check the ovaries and tubes, can in many cases lend certainty to an ambiguous diagnosis before the tube ruptures (see Figure 24).

☐ *The treatment of ectopic pregnancy* depends on the size of the embryo at the time of diagnosis. The most common approach to ruptured or unruptured tubal pregnancies, *if* the woman has a normal second tube, is the total removal of the tube, a "salpingectomy." If a tubal pregnancy occurs in a woman with only one remaining tube the doctor will try, if possible, to save the tube so it can be repaired (either during the same operation or at a later date). If the tube is unruptured, it may be possible, for example, for the pregnancy to be "milked" out of the open fimbrial end of the tube. If no excessive bleeding results, further surgery may not be necessary. If the abnormal pregnancy is in the middle of an unruptured tube it may be possible to slice open the tube, ease out the pregnancy, and stitch the tube back up; or, perhaps, remove the segment of tube containing the pregnancy and sew the loose ends together. Rh immunoglobulin should also be given to Rh-negative women with ectopic pregnancies.

The woman who has had an ectopic pregnancy, even if her other tube seems to be normal, has an increased risk of another ectopic pregnancy—perhaps as high as 10 to 15 in 100, compared to the normal woman's one in 100. However, the good news is that 50 percent of women who have had an ectopic pregnancy will go on to successfully bear a child.

20

Prenatal Testing

One of the most exciting advances in all of medicine during the last few decades has been our new ability to evaluate the health of the fetus while it's still snug in the uterus. Before these new tests were developed, we really couldn't tell much about what was going on in the fetus's small self-contained world. We could listen to its heartbeat with a stethoscope, roughly estimate its size and age by feeling the expanding uterus within the abdomen, and, if necessary, use various types of x-rays to determine the fetus's developmental stage and viability.

As I write, a wide range of tests have been developed which can reveal much about the fetus at many different stages of pregnancy. And these tests are continually being improved—made faster, safer, more accurate. Genetic defects can sometimes be diagnosed in the uterus, as can some developmental problems of the brain and spine, Rh disease of pregnancy (a mother/fetus blood incompatibility problem), intrauterine growth retardation (slowed fetal growth), and much, much more.

Of course, keeping an eye on fetal health is important in *every* pregnancy. Obstetricians have divided certain pregnancies into "high-risk" groups so that special attention, including the above tests, can be given in situations in which the baby is clearly at increased risk. Women with these conditions can then be given special vigilance throughout pregnancy and labor so any problems can be taken care of swiftly, efficiently, and with the least harm possible to mother and child.

Although "high risk" has been defined in various ways, the following is a list of conditions which I feel place a woman in a category requiring special care. This doesn't mean something *will* go wrong. In fact, it probably won't. But since the chances here of a problem are higher than in women who don't fall into one of these groups, it's wise for women, their partners, and their doctors to be prepared, just in case.

- maternal age over thirty-five
- maternal age under eighteen
- anemia
- high blood pressure
- diabetes
- obesity
- malnutrition
- previous cesarean section
- past obstetrical problem (such as miscarriage, prematurity, or still-birth)
- infections (kidney, liver; viral, bacterial, etc.)
- fibroid tumors of the uterus
- cancer
- epilepsy
- family history of genetic disease

The techniques that allow us to measure fetal health, all of which will be explained later, include alpha-fetoprotein testing, amniocentesis, chorionic villous sampling, electronic fetal monitoring, fetal blood sampling, and ultrasonography.

ALPHA-FETOPROTEIN TESTING

A new test of the mother's blood, called the "alpha-fetoprotein" (AFP) test, helps to single out the small number of women whose unborn babies may have a problem called a "neural tube defect." It also offers the remaining majority of women the reassurance that, once their test comes back normal, their babies are not likely to have this serious brain or spinal cord problem.

Neural tube defects are so named because the central nervous system—the brain and the spinal cord—develop from a structure in the embryo called the "neural tube." Normally, the neural tube closes completely. However, if it fails to close, it may leave a defect, or opening, somewhere along the central nervous system. In some cases the opening in the spinal cord may be covered with bone and skin (this is a closed neural tube defect); in others it may be completely uncovered (an open neural tube defect). Two common and serious types of neural tube defects are anencephaly and spina bifida. Anencephaly occurs when the brain and skull do not develop normally. Such a fetus cannot survive. In spina bifida, the opening is in the spinal cord, a problem that varies from somewhat minor to very serious depending on its type and location.

Alpha-fetoprotein (AFP) is a substance produced by the fetus. If the neural tube is not closed, large amounts of AFP can spill into the amniotic fluid and, from there, into the mother's blood. Measurement of the mother's blood and amniotic fluid for AFP can detect elevated levels that may be due to a neural tube defect.

Your physician will draw a blood sample between sixteen and nineteen weeks of pregnancy to test for AFP. If that shows elevated levels, the test will be repeated immediately. If your blood test has normal levels of AFP, there is no need for further tests. However, the test is not infallible. The first AFP test may miss as much as 20 percent of neural tube defects.

If the second test is also elevated, there is still only about a 4–10 percent chance that the fetus actually has an open neural tube defect. Other things can elevate AFP levels: twins, for example, or a pregnancy more advanced than previously suspected. Therefore, after two high AFP levels, additional tests will be performed to determine the cause. Sonography, or ultrasound, already referred to several times, is used to correctly date the pregnancy and rule out twins. If no obvious defect is seen on ultrasound, dates appear correct, and twins are ruled out, amniocentesis (more on this later) is the next step.

If amniocentesis detects a high AFP level in the amniotic fluid, the fetus is very likely to have a neural tube defect. Another enzyme called "acetylcholinesterase" can also be measured in the amniotic fluid to add certainty to the diagnosis. High-resolution sonography (a more advanced and accurate type of ultrasound exam) should be done to search for the defect. At that point a couple may be faced with the difficult decision of whether or not to continue the pregnancy (see Table 8).

The cause of neural tube defects is not known. Genetic and environmental factors (including diet) may play a part, but no one really

TABLE 8

Blood drawn all pregnant women 16–19 weeks if no
amniocentesis is to be performed

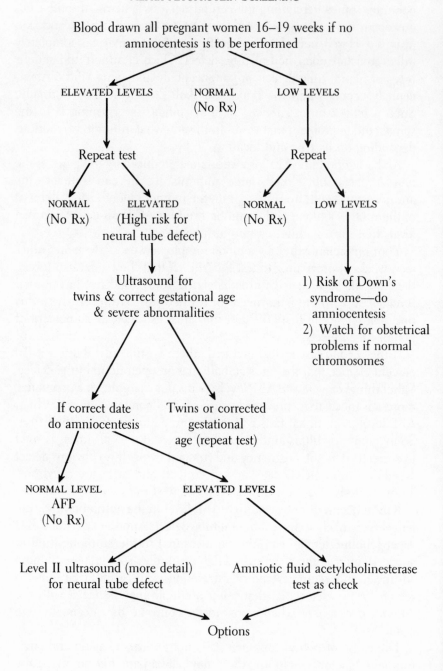

ELEVATED LEVELS   NORMAL   LOW LEVELS
(No Rx)

Repeat test   Repeat

NORMAL   ELEVATED   NORMAL   LOW LEVELS
(No Rx)   (High risk for   (No Rx)
         neural tube defect)

Ultrasound for
twins & correct gestational age
& severe abnormalities

1) Risk of Down's
syndrome—do
amniocentesis
2) Watch for obstetrical
problems if normal
chromosomes

If correct date   Twins or corrected
do amniocentesis   gestational
            age (repeat test)

NORMAL LEVEL   ELEVATED LEVELS
AFP
(No Rx)

Level II ultrasound (more detail)   Amniotic fluid acetylcholinesterase
for neural tube defect   test as check

Options

knows for sure. In the United States, one to two live births per 1,000 involve a neural tube defect, half of which are spina bifida. Most occur in couples with no special risks. However, risks are increased in women who have had a child with a neural tube defect and in couples in which one partner has a neural tube defect or a family history of a neural tube defect. Your physician can counsel you on the cost, special risks, and availability of this test.

ULTRASOUND

Sonography or "ultrasound" is probably the single most successful method of intrauterine diagnosis that has evolved in recent years. A variation on ultrasound—called "sonar"—was used during World War II to scout out submarines lurking deep in the oceans. After that, "sonar" began to show its strengths in medicine. Recent technological advances have raised picture quality from "merely" remarkable (i.e., a trained technician could translate the blurry black and white lines and blobs into a recognizable baby) to simply amazing (so clear, doctors and mothers gaze in wonder together at the absolutely unmistakable humanity of the tiny form). "From the second I saw our baby on the scanner, she was real in a way that had not struck me before, for all the pregnancy tests and doctors' visits," one woman told me. "She was no longer a fetus, she was my child. My husband was just as bowled over as I." Ultrasound has enhanced almost beyond measure our ability to evaluate the health of the fetus, with no known risk at this time. No x-rays, no needles, no pain.

The "magic" is in the method of ultrasound: sound waves of high frequency, above the range of human hearing. Sound is a physical force that is in no way related to x-ray. Therefore, it does not have any of the tissue-harming potential of x-ray exposure during pregnancy. These sound waves are sent out by a scanner, or a "transducer," held over the abdomen, and travel into the body as vibrations. Echoes from the sound waves are reflected off the various surfaces within the body as the waves pass through—a fetus in the uterus, fluid, bone, tissue, organs. The echoes are translated into electrical signals that, when projected onto a TV-like screen, reveal a detailed picture of these normally hidden structures.

Ultrasound is used in a number of ways. It can measure size, such as the bones in the fetus's arms or head. It can identify the shape and location of structures like the uterus and placenta. Movements, such as the fetal heart beating, can be seen, and still photographs can be made to record permanently what was revealed.

During pregnancy, ultrasound can be used in many specific ways:

- Pregnancy can be confirmed. The fetal sac can be seen in the uterus as early as three weeks after conception;
- The fetus can be proven to be alive, by demonstration of its beating heart, as early as seven or eight weeks from the last menstrual period;
- Multiple births—twins, most often—can be identified with accuracy by the third month;
- The width of the fetal skull and the length of the femur bones in the legs can reveal the age of the fetus, so due dates can be checked. Several scans of these bones over time can determine if the fetus is growing normally;
- Major physical abnormalities (of kidneys, intestines, limbs, or spine, for example) can be visualized;
- The placenta can be scanned for clues to the cause of abnormal bleeding;
- Problems with the amount of amniotic fluid (polyhydramnios is too much; oligohydramnios is too little) can be diagnosed;
- Fibroid tumors of the uterus and ovarian masses can be tracked during pregnancy;
- Rare placental pregnancies, such as molar pregnancies (a rare placental tumor), can be diagnosed;
- A "biophysical profile" of the fetus can be done to measure its overall well-being. This profile includes fetal movements, fetal muscle tone, the amount of amniotic fluid, and fetal breathing movements.

Concern about the possible long-term effects of ultrasound on the fetus has been raised. No damage has been documented to a single mother or fetus after twenty years of ultrasound use in medical centers throughout the world; however, since even this extensive use leaves sonography still categorized as a relatively new procedure, it should be used only when there is a medical need for it, not simply out of curiosity. If the examination is needed to diagnose or rule out a suspected problem, almost every obstetrician would agree that the very real benefits obtained from this test outweigh a risk that is purely theoretical at this time.

☐ *Having an ultrasound* may involve your physician's asking you to have a full bladder during this examination (see Figures 20 and 21). This may make you somewhat uncomfortable but does make the results clearer. Otherwise, the procedure does not entail any discomfort—no needles, drugs, or special diet are required. The examination is performed by either your physician or a trained ultrasound technician in a hospital or an office. You will lie on your back on an examination table. An oily substance will be rubbed on the skin of your abdomen so that the transducer can slide across it easily and smoothly. The oil also improves the penetration of the sound waves into your body by "sealing" the transducer to your skin and eliminating any air pockets between the two.

The exam itself will take less than 30 minutes. The image of the fetus will be visible on a TV screen, and still pictures may be taken of the screen image at various points. The sonographer may be able to tell you the baby's sex, if you want to know it before birth. Bonding, which normally occurs between parents and newborn just after birth, may also occur to some extent even before birth once ultrasound reveals your tiny offspring swimming and kicking in its little underwater world.

AMNIOCENTESIS

Amniocentesis has become one of the major tools of the perinatologist. Although it sounds frightening, and is a bit disconcerting to undergo, it is generally safe and simple in the hands of an expert. Amniocentesis is performed by passing a long, thin needle straight through the skin of the abdomen and the uterine wall and into the amniotic sac—the structure that holds the fetus and its protective fluid "swimming pool" (see Figure 22). A small portion of the amniotic fluid is then sucked up into the needle, to be studied in various ways. "I was pretty scared about the thought of that needle," one apprehensive mother told me, echoing the sentiments of many others. "But," she added (as women almost always do), "although I could feel an odd kind of pressure, it wasn't really uncomfortable or painful."

Amniocentesis is quite safe. It's done after sixteen weeks (once sufficient fluid has formed) either in the office or in a hospital, depending on where the ultrasound equipment is. The location of the fetus and placenta is determined by ultrasound so that they will not be harmed by a stray poke of the needle. However, as with any medical procedure, the risks of the amniocentesis should be weighed against the seriousness of the potential problem it is being done to detect. Minor complications

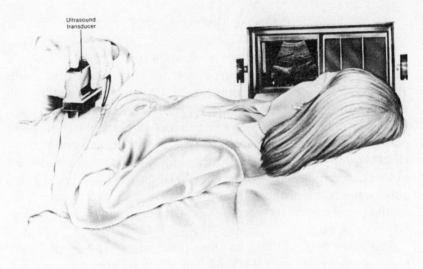

FIGURE 20

Ultrasound technique
Courtesy of Syntex Laboratories, Inc.

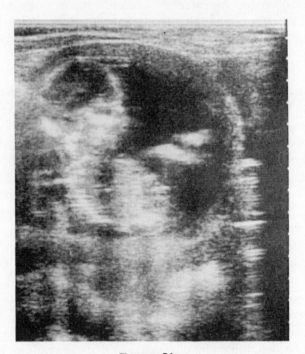

FIGURE 21

Ultrasound picture of 10–11-week fetus

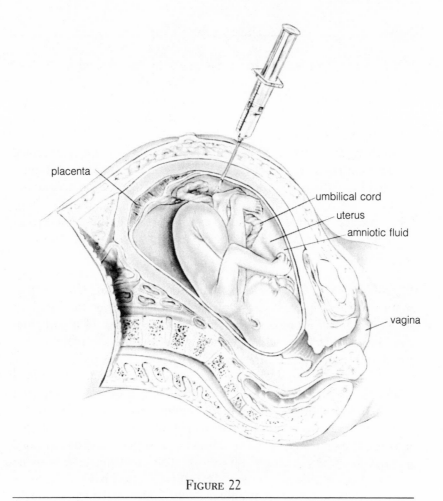

placenta

umbilical cord
uterus
amniotic fluid

vagina

FIGURE 22

Amniocentesis
Courtesy of Syntex Laboratories, Inc.

for the mother include cramping, bleeding, and leakage of amniotic fluid. Fortunately, these problems occur in fewer than one in 400 cases and they usually require no treatment. Serious complications of amniocentesis, such as miscarriage and fetal injury, occur very infrequently, in fewer than one in 600 cases. Women with Rh-negative blood require Rh immunoglobulin after the procedure, to prevent Rh sensitization (see Chapter 21, "Medical Problems in Pregnancy").

The following are some of the most common reasons amniocentesis is used:

□ *Rh disease* frequency has been markedly diminished by the development of the immune vaccine that keeps the Rh-negative mother from *ever* developing the antibodies harmful to her Rh-positive fetuses. Tests such as amniocentesis can greatly aid in the care of those few cases that still do occur.

Studying the amniotic fluid of an Rh-sensitized woman (as explained in the next chapter) enables a physician to determine how seriously affected the fetus is. The levels of bilirubin, a sign of the destruction of the fetus's red blood cells, can be measured in the amniotic fluid. The degree of anemia of the fetus can then be determined and treatment given if necessary. The test is also used to determine the optimum time for delivery.

□ *Respiratory distress syndrome* is a lung condition of many premature infants that can cause death because it leaves the newborn unable to breathe properly. It is caused by the lack of a particular substance, surfactant, which normally forms on the surface of the lungs and facilitates the exchange of oxygen and carbon dioxide. The cause of hyaline membrane disease (an older name for respiratory distress syndrome) is not well understood, but it develops only after birth and does not occur *in utero*. Amniotic fluid can be tested for the presence of surfactant in order to zero in on which babies could develop the disease if delivered too soon. This may be necessary in complicated pregnancies when a decision has to be made whether to deliver the fetus or hold off a while longer. The surfactant test has proven to be very accurate and has greatly enhanced the ability of the perinatologist to make the best decisions about high-risk pregnancies. It is also used many times prior to performing a nonemergency cesarean section, to make sure that the fetus's lungs are mature.

□ *Diagnosing birth defects* owes much to amniocentesis, which has become a valuable tool in—and is probably best known for—the prenatal diagnosis of birth defects. This now-well-established procedure is critical to diagnosing the presence or absence of over 100 different chromosomal abnormalities. Genetic amniocentesis may be done if either parent or a previous child has chromosome abnormalities, if the mother is thirty-five years old or over or has had a child with Down's syndrome, if the parents are carriers of sex-linked diseases such as hemophilia or of autosomal recessive diseases such as Tay-Sachs disease, or if a neural tube defect is suspected (see Chapter 14, "Genetic Counseling," for more information).

CHORIONIC VILLOUS SAMPLING: THE NEXT STEP?

Although amniocentesis has proven extraordinarily valuable, it does have several limitations. One is that the procedure cannot be done before sixteen weeks of pregnancy and often requires a three- to four-week wait for the results. Therefore, it may not be until 20 weeks of pregnancy—the fifth month—before a woman gets the results. If termination of the pregnancy is then elected because of fetal abnormalities, it is much more traumatic at this point, both psychologically and medically. Therefore, if there were a safe and reliable test for diagnosing fetal problems early—during the first trimester—it would be of enormous value.

One such technique, called "chorionic villous biopsy" or "chorionic villous sampling" (CVS), looks quite promising at the moment. Using ultrasound as a guide, it is possible to pass a small tube into the uterus through the cervix at about 11 weeks of pregnancy. A tiny bit of tissue from the layer of the placenta known as the "chorion" can be drawn into the tube and removed for study. (Ultrasound will also be done before the test to confirm the presence of a good, healthy fetal heartbeat. If there is no heartbeat by 10 to 11 weeks it usually means that the woman is going to have a miscarriage and is, therefore, not a candidate for the chorionic villous biopsy.)

The small chunk of tissue taken from the chorion can be used for chromosomal studies directly—without waiting to grow the tissue in culture, as is necessary with amniocentesis. Therefore, results of genetic studies can be available just 24 to 48 hours after sampling. Just about every disorder that can be found with amniocentesis can be diagnosed by CVS much earlier (except neural tube defects, which are diagnosable by amniocentesis and alpha-fetoprotein tests).

However, CVS still must be considered experimental as I write this book. One of the major problems at this point is the risk of miscarriage. Most studies show a spontaneous abortion rate of 1 to 3 percent above the usual rate. At this time women who have a relatively low risk of having a baby with detectable defects are discouraged from having CVS and encouraged to have amniocentesis. However, in very-high-risk situations the risk of miscarriage may be considered worth taking.

As of this date some 4,000 women have undergone testing by this new technique. Undoubtedly, much more will be learned about how to make it safer.

Another prenatal use of this procedure will be by couples deciding to have a child of a particular sex. Let's say there's a family history of a disorder like hemophilia, which would affect only male fetuses. CVS could determine the fetus's sex early, still timely for an early abortion. Of course, if this were possible, parents would also have the ability to abort a child for reasons of sexual preference alone—if, for example, they had three boys and wanted a girl. This raises difficult ethical questions for both patients and physicians.

FETOSCOPY: BLOOD SAMPLES AND FETAL SIGHTINGS

Another technique still in the promising but risky experimental stage is called "fetoscopy." This technique involves the use of a viewing instrument passed through the abdomen and into the amniotic sac. This allows the physician to look directly at the fetus and the placenta, and sample the fetus's blood, from which every major detectable genetic disorder can be accurately diagnosed. However, this procedure has high risks and limitations that haven't been ironed out and is, therefore, still done only at major medical centers and regarded as experimental.

FETAL MONITORING: CLUES FROM THE HEART

It has been known for years that the fetus's heart rate changes in certain situations. But only recently has technology evolved to where these changes can be measured and interpreted. Today the fetal heart rate is sometimes checked during pregnancy with an "antepartum non-stress test," and during labor, with two different techniques—external and internal monitoring.

High-risk pregnancies can be monitored during the pregnancy with the antepartum non-stress test. This test is based on the physiologic fact that the healthy fetus's heart beats faster when it moves—much as yours does when you run up a flight of stairs. The absence of a heart rate speed-up during fetal movement may indicate the fetus is in trouble. This test is done with a heart rate monitor strapped to the mother's belly and may be performed in the office. When she feels a wiggle from the fetus, she indicates this, and it is correlated with the heart rate. If the non-stress test suggests that the fetus is having some difficulty, there are further tests that will probably be done to evaluate its condition more precisely.

Fetal monitoring during labor has become routine in many medical centers. This is done with two belts strapped around the woman's abdomen, each holding a transducer (a measuring device). One charts the fetal heart rate and pattern and the other marks the frequency and duration of the uterine contractions. As with the non-stress test, it's the comparison of two things that is important. Here, it's how the fetal heart rate correlates with uterine contractions (instead of with fetal movement, as in the non-stress test). Heart rates may slow, speed up, or alter their patterns with stress. We can now detect very subtle alterations of the fetal heart rate in association with uterine contractions, so that a fetus in trouble can be spotted quickly. There is no question that fetal monitoring has saved the lives of infants whose difficulties would otherwise have been unsuspected until, perhaps, too late. However, its *routine* use in all labor is still being debated.

Another test, called "fetal scalp blood sampling," can also be done during labor to determine whether the fetus is being unduly stressed by the birth process. Once the cervix is partially dilated a device may be slipped in to obtain a few drops of blood from the fetus's scalp. The blood can then be measured for its acid base balance, or pH. A drop in pH to below 7.2 signals that the fetus is having distress and requires immediate delivery, by cesarean section if necessary.

The combination of fetal heart rate monitoring and fetal blood sampling during labor has proven highly accurate in diagnosing fetal distress and determining which fetuses should be delivered immediately. By treating fetal distress the chances of severe injury and permanent damage (such as cerebral palsy) can be reduced.

In summary, the development of these tests for keeping track of the fetus's health while it's still in the uterus has truly made the concept of "two patients"—the fetus and the mother—a reality. Both can be evaluated, both cared for, and both receive the benefits of high-level health care. No longer are obstetricians concerned with just delivering a baby. We now have the means to act on our concern that a child be born as safely as possible and in the best possible condition. This is truly a satisfying, exciting, and challenging time to be an obstetrician.

21

Medical Problems in Pregnancy

Pregnancy is a unique condition in two very distinct ways. First, it has an intense impact on women's minds and bodies over a precisely specified period of time. Second, it is the only condition in which the needs and interests of two patients—mother and fetus—are so completely intertwined. Any health problem a pregnant woman may have has the potential to affect her baby, before or after birth. The purpose of this chapter is to briefly outline some of the most common medical problems that may affect pregnancy, so that women with these conditions can plan their pregnancies with information and intelligence. I won't relate all the details of care in each case—that is for each woman to go over with her physician—but I will give a general overview of how the conditions discussed below tend to affect pregnancy.

DIABETES

Before insulin became available in 1922, diabetic women and their unborn children had a very good chance of dying during pregnancy. Once insulin came into widespread use, death rates among pregnant diabetics fell immediately and dramatically, but their babies still had a very rough time. Only in the past five years or so has infant health markedly improved. There are many reasons for this, including fetal monitoring, the development of ultrasound, the establishment of newborn intensive-care units, and, most importantly, further improvements in the care of the pregnant diabetic.

We now know that many of the problems seen in the infants of diabetic mothers are caused by high glucose levels in the mother's blood. If blood sugar can be controlled during the early months of pregnancy, babies will have fewer congenital abnormalities, less chance of being overly large and sick, and, quite simply, more of a chance to be healthier overall.

A diabetic woman's pregnancy must be carefully planned so that optimum diabetic control can be established *before* conception. She will be closely monitored for insulin and blood sugar levels. General principles of good health and hygiene and knowledge of pregnancy's health hazards are even more vital to the diabetic woman, and will be stressed by her doctor during the planning-for-pregnancy stages. It is also important that such women know that their chances of having a diabetic child are very small—only about one in 100. If *both* parents are diabetic the chances rise to about 5 in 100. This need not be a major concern in a diabetic couple's discussions about having a child.

The marked improvement in dealing with the pregnancies of diabetic women is one of the major advances in obstetrical care in the past ten years. But prepregnancy counseling and management are a critical part of this success. The pregnant diabetic should enter pregnancy with the knowledge, ability, and desire to achieve maximum results.

Within the scope of this book it is not possible to outline in detail the management of diabetic pregnancies—which includes maintenance of low blood sugar, strict diet control, and tests to assess the fetus's health—but it must simply be stressed that if you are in this situation, you need a doctor experienced in diabetic pregnancies; there are such specialists available, and planning and knowledge are of utmost importance to you.

OBESITY

Obesity affects in two ways a woman's ability to reproduce. First, many very heavy women fail to ovulate at all until a critical amount of weight has been lost. Second, obesity during pregnancy means a woman has a much higher chance of developing high blood pressure and abnormal blood sugar metabolism, or latent diabetes. Extremely large babies are also more common, which can lead to difficult deliveries. And the cesarean rate is also slightly higher.

While pregnancies in very overweight women require special

care, things tend to go quite well when the situation is appropriately managed. Weight reduction is very successful in inducing ovulation in previously infertile women, and is, for general health reasons, the best course to pursue even with fertile obese women. Significant weight reduction *during* pregnancy is not possible, so for the best, healthiest pregnancy as much weight as possible should be lost before conception.

Heart Disease and Pregnancy

The care and management of pregnant women with heart disease (such as congenital heart disease and rheumatic heart disease) has also improved significantly due to advances in the management of the disease itself, the development of antibiotics (to prevent the heart infections which are more common in these women), and to advances in prenatal testing. It is now possible for virtually any woman with heart disease, except those with the most advanced cases, to carry a pregnancy successfully.

Here, too, one of the cornerstones of management is prepregnancy counseling and an active program of care during pregnancy. Avoiding infection, taking the appropriate medications, and watching the diet are all very important. Hospitalization may be necessary at critical periods to reduce the risks to the mother and enhance the chances of the fetus staying healthy. There pregnancies require expert management. A woman with heart disease *must* receive medical counseling from someone with experience in this area before she becomes pregnant.

Rh Disease of Pregnancy

Rh disease (in which, basically, antibodies in the mother's blood destroy the fetus's red blood cells) has become much less common since the development of Rh vaccination—a shot of immunoglobulin given after first pregnancies, whether they be abortions, miscarriages, ectopics, or normal term deliveries.

Rh disease occurs when a woman with Rh-negative blood carries an Rh-positive fetus. During the pregnancy or following abortion or delivery some of the fetus's red blood cells can pass through the placenta into the mother's circulation and produce an antibody response to the foreign red cells in her body. (The "Rh factor" is located in the red blood cells.) The woman is now said to be "sensitized" to Rh factor: The antibodies in her blood will respond to Rh-positive blood as if it were an invader—just as if it were a harmful bacteria or deadly virus. During a later pregnancy with an Rh-positive fetus, these antibodies in the mother's blood can pass back through the placenta into the new fetus, and attack and destroy that fetus's red blood cells. This produces anemia in the fetus and severe illness, even death. Fortunately, the use of Rh immunoglobulin has reduced the incidence of this disease in susceptible women to fewer than 3 in 1,000 pregnancies.

It is important that all pregnant women have their blood type checked (this is a routine part of most obstetricians' prenatal care). Rh-negative women delivering an Rh-positive fetus should be given an injection of Rh immunoglobulin within 72 hours of delivery to keep them from making antibodies. All Rh-negative women who have miscarriages or abortions should also have the vaccination. In addition, when a pregnant Rh-negative woman undergoes the prenatal test called "amniocentesis," she should receive an Rh vaccination as well.

Recently it has become routine in most medical centers to give Rh immunoglobulin to every Rh-negative woman at 28 weeks of pregnancy. This use at 28 weeks prevents the rare sensitization case that occurs during a pregnancy and affects that fetus.

Table 9 summarizes the indications for the use of Rh immunoglobulin in pregnancy. Adopting this actively preventive program of Rh immunization could wipe out virtually 100 percent of Rh disease.

The care of women who do become sensitized to Rh factor prior to vaccination (or for any other reason) has also made great advances. Amniocentesis will check the baby's health in the uterus. If necessary, the newborn can receive transfusions immediately after birth; and great strides have been made in actually giving a life-saving blood transfusion in severe cases to a fetus in the womb. These techniques have markedly reduced the chances of fetal death from this disease.

The conquest of Rh disease is one of the major success stories of modern obstetrics.

INFECTION DURING PREGNANCY

The pregnant woman, just like her nonpregnant peers, may catch infections of the urinary tract, lungs, or any other organ system. By

TABLE 9

NEED AND USE OF RH IMMUNOGLOBULIN IN PREGNANCY

1ST TRIMESTER
    Abortions (spontaneous or induced)
    Ectopic pregnancy

2ND TRIMESTER
    Amniocentesis
    Late abortion
    Premature delivery
    Routine use at 28 weeks in all Rh-negative women
    Bleeding episode

3RD TRIMESTER
    After normal delivery by any method
    Amniocentesis
    Bleeding episode prior to delivery

NOTE: With abruptio placentae (placenta separates from uterine wall before the baby is born), placenta previa (the placenta covers the cervix so it's between baby's head and the outside world), bleeding episodes, or difficult delivery, extra amounts of Rh immunoglobulin may need to be administered. This can be decided by examining the number of fetal cells in the mother's blood after the above events.

and large, these infections are well tolerated by mother and baby and are treated in the same way as in the nonpregnant woman.

However, some infections, especially the viral ones, can harm the fetus. The giving of vaccinations before and during pregnancy is outlined in Chapter 17, "Prenatal Care," and careful prepregnancy counseling in light of those recommendations can help avert some potential tragedies during pregnancy.

The use of most antibiotics is permissible during pregnancy to treat the various bacterial infections that may attack women. Local infections of the vagina, such as yeast, trichomonas, and hemophilus, can be treated locally without difficulty during pregnancy. However, antibiotics can kill only bacteria but not viruses, so there is no real treatment for most viral infections. Some viruses, such as rubella (German measles) and primary herpes, can have grave consequences for the fetus, including death or malformations.

One of the major principles in the management of infections in pregnant women is to avoid fevers. High fever, all by itself, can cause premature labor. It is important that a pregnant woman with any fever-causing illness take, on her doctor's advice, appropriate medication such as Tylenol to bring down the temperature.

Hepatitis, a viral infection, comes in two varieties, type A and type B. Hepatitis A, the milder form, is not transmitted to the fetus and, therefore, poses no risk during pregnancy. However, pregnant women exposed to hepatitis A should be given serum gammaglobulin, which affords some protection against contracting the disease. The newborn, unlike the sheltered fetus, is at risk for acquiring the disease from its infected mother. Infants, then, should be given gammaglobulin within two weeks of delivery.

With hepatitis B (serum type) the risk of fetal infection is 75 percent in women who come down with the disease during the last trimester of pregnancy. Infants are at risk for the first two months postpartum. Early in pregnancy there is much less risk to the fetus. Hepatitis B immunoglobulin should be given at birth to children of women who are either chronic carriers of hepatitis B or who have an acute infection. If the mother is a carrier, this should be followed by vaccination against hepatitis B at three months of age.

THROMBOPHLEBITIS

The risk of forming blood clots in the legs (thrombophlebitis), which can then travel to the lungs and cause a pulmonary embolism (lung clot) and death, is higher than normal during pregnancy and just after. This is due to the increased capacity of blood to clot during pregnancy and the pooling of blood in the legs. Women who deliver by cesarean section are especially at risk. Fast, accurate diagnosis is of utmost importance in this potentially serious disorder.

Women who have had severe thrombophlebitis or a pulmonary embolus (lung clot) before they became pregnant may need to take anticoagulants—drugs that inhibit blood's clotting—during pregnancy. The only drug that can safely be used is one called "heparin," since it does not cross the placenta into the fetus. Drugs such as Coumadin derivatives should never be used; they do cross the placenta and can produce hemorrhages in the fetus. After birth, heparin may be used to prevent more clots and Coumadin may be used for six to eight months. Although heparin must be given by injection, women often become adept at giving themselves doses of the drug.

HIGH BLOOD PRESSURE

Hypertension in pregnancy can be managed quite handily with the modern drug arsenal now available to doctors. If blood pressure is not kept down to normal levels during pregnancy there is a risk that the fetus will not grow properly (intrauterine growth retardation, IUGR), that it may be born too soon (prematurity), or even be born dead (stillborn). By careful use of medication the blood pressure can be controlled so that the placenta can function normally and the fetus can grow and thrive.

Women with hypertension are at risk for toxemia of pregnancy and must be followed closely. Toxemia is a syndrome in pregnancy characterized by high blood pressure, edema (fluid accumulation), and protein in the urine. It appears more commonly in women who had high blood pressure before pregnancy. All the modern techniques of fetal monitoring and fetal testing (including ultrasound and other tests described in Chapter 20, "Prenatal Testing") are called upon to track the health of mother and child. With their help, the chances of a healthy baby, safely born, are good.

RENAL DISEASE

Urinary tract infections are among the most common women can get, as I explained in Chapter 7, "Common Infections." Frequent bouts with cystitis (bladder infections) and even occasional kidney infections do not keep women from becoming pregnant.

However, urinary tract infections during pregnancy are associated with a higher risk of premature delivery and slowed fetal growth. Therefore, women prone to urinary tract infections must be alert to their symptoms, and their doctors should do urinary tract cultures at least twice during the pregnancy. If any signs of trouble appear, antibiotics can be given to nip the problem in the bud. Kept under control, urinary tract infections should not cause a woman to worry.

GASTROINTESTINAL DISORDERS

Inflammatory bowel disease (ileitis and colitis) are difficult health problems for the young women who have them. But many significant advances have kept these diseases under control—including the use of steroids, antimetabolites, and antibiotics.

For the best chance of a healthy pregnancy, it is generally recommended that women with these disorders wait for a remission for one year before they try to get pregnant. However, about one-third of them will have a recurrence anyway, either early in the pregnancy or just after. Steroids and antibiotics can be safely used during pregnancy if this happens. Women who have had ileostomies or colostomies (operations in which part of the intestines are removed, leaving a hole in the abdomen through which stool passes into a bag) can also have normal pregnancies and normal deliveries with good obstetrical care.

For more information on the impact of these diseases on pregnancy, you can write to the National Foundation for Ileitis and Colitis at 295 Madison Avenue, Suite 519, New York, N.Y. 10017.

GALL BLADDER DISEASE

Pregnancy itself makes gall bladder disease and stones in the bile tract more likely. This is because the bile organs work more sluggishly during pregnancy, allowing elevated levels of cholesterol in the bloodstream. Women with this problem, especially if they have known stones, should try to have them treated before becoming pregnant. This usually requires surgery. During pregnancy, attacks of gall bladder disease can be treated without harming the fetus, but a low-fat diet should be adhered to, to lower the chances of a problem. It is rare for surgery to be required for acute episodes of this disease during pregnancy, but it can be done successfully if necessary.

ANEMIA

There are major changes in the blood during pregnancy, due to the demands of both placenta and fetus, that cause an increased need for iron. Women who start pregnancy with an iron deficiency or anemia place both themselves and their babies at a disadvantage.

When iron is in short supply, however, the fetus tends to get its iron any way it can—which, of course, comes down to hogging the mother's supply, increasing her anemia. Severe anemia in pregnant women may slow fetal growth and cause premature delivery. The most common cause of anemia in pregnancy, iron deficiency, occurs in 15 to 50 percent of pregnant women in the United States. Iron deficiency during pregnancy can be prevented by taking 30 to 60 milligrams of iron daily. A blood check for anemia before pregnancy allows any deficiency to be corrected, so that women won't be facing an uphill battle for the next nine months.

EPILEPSY

In general, women with epilepsy do well during pregnancy. Although no one knows why, the frequency of seizures has been reported to increase in 25 percent of pregnant women, decrease in another 25 percent, and stay the same as before half the time.

The major issue for the pregnant epileptic is that of the safety of the drugs she takes to prevent seizures. Some of them, such as hydantoins, are definitely associated with an increased risk of birth defects. Children born to epileptic mothers not taking drugs have a 2.3 percent incidence of congenital malformations (which is higher than normal), whereas those receiving antiepilepsy drugs have as high as an 11.5 percent risk.

Women with epilepsy should be advised before pregnancy about the risk of birth defects. Excessive weight gain and fluid retention during pregnancy should be avoided. If the woman is on drug therapy, the use of a single drug rather than multiples is best. Phenobarbital is probably the most desirable, since it appears to be the safest antiseizure drug available.

BREAST DISEASE DURING PREGNANCY

The breasts undergo marked changes during pregnancy. The glands enlarge rapidly—the effect of pregnancy hormones to prepare a woman for breastfeeding. Benign diseases of the breast are much more common during pregnancy than breast cancer, just as in nonpregnant women. But they do not generally present a serious risk to the mother or the fetus.

Between 10 and 25 percent of breast cancers occur during the reproductive years, so some of those are bound to be in pregnant women.

It has been estimated that between 1,000 and 2,000 pregnant women per year will have breast cancer: That's about 2 per 10,000 pregnancies in the United States. Most of these masses will be found by the woman herself. However, all women should have a thorough breast examination as part of their first physical examination during pregnancy.

When a suspicious mass is found, a biopsy (surgical sampling of the lump for examination under a microscope) will be required for a firm diagnosis. Generally, treatment of malignant lesions during pregnancy is the same as for nonpregnant women, with some changed procedures. How successful treatment is at this time is somewhat unclear. Studies suggest that most of the poor outcomes are due to delays in diagnosis and treatment rather than to any difference in the nature of the disease itself. As of now, there is no evidence that termination of the pregnancy will help in the treatment. However, chemotherapy must be withheld, especially during the first 12 weeks of pregnancy because of its teratogenic (birth-defect-producing) potential. Radiation therapy should be postponed if the woman is close to delivery, although there is no consensus as to how close. Early in pregnancy, when the risks to the woman of delaying would increase too much for her to wait until birth, radiation can be given as long as a lead shield is placed over the woman's abdomen and pelvis to protect the fetus.

Pregnancy after breast cancer treatment is another subject which has seen some controversy. It used to be felt that women should delay pregnancy for two to five years after treatment, because of the fear that pregnancy would activate the disease. However, at the current time opinion varies but can be best summarized as follows: Women who have been treated recently for breast cancer should probably wait awhile before becoming pregnant, since there seems to be a higher chance of treatment failure if pregnancy follows too closely; however, after a number of years there is no definite evidence that pregnancy will increase the chance of cancer recurrence. Discuss this with your physician.

☐ *Breast cancer and lactation*   present another kind of problem. Diagnosis of breast cancer in a lactating woman who is breastfeeding is difficult since, just as in pregnancy, the breast is larger than normal, and may have small lumps and bumps. However, it is just as important that any suspicious mass be biopsied so that there will be no delay in diagnosis if cancer is found. If this occurs, breastfeeding must be discontinued and the appropriate therapy begun.

Women who have had cancer in one breast may breastfeed from the other. There is also no evidence to support the fear that breastfeeding increases the risk of the baby someday developing breast cancer through the spread of a virus. It appears most likely that genetics, rather than a virus, is the link to the increased risk of breast cancer in the daughters of women with this disease.

PREGNANCY AFTER DES EXPOSURE

From the late 1940s to the 1970s an estimated two to three million women were given diethylstilbestrol (DES) during their pregnancies to prevent miscarriages. Continuing studies on the drug showed that DES didn't seem to work in treating the disorders for which it was prescribed, so doctors stopped using it. At the time, between one million and one and a half million babies had been exposed to the drug in the uterus.

Eventually, the long-term consequences of this exposure started to come to light. Cancer of the vagina in seven girls was first reported in 1970. These seven cases alerted the medical world to the link between this normally quite rare cancer and *in utero* DES exposure, and the terrible irony of this drug—given to try to save pregnancies—became clear. The legacy of DES exposure has continued to expand since then and even includes fertility problems in men. Although new cases of vaginal carcinoma seem to be becoming less frequent, "DES babies" have now entered their own reproductive years, and new problems have come to light:

• The risk of spontaneous abortions (miscarriages) is approximately twice as high in DES-exposed women as in unexposed women.
• Premature delivery is approximately three times as common as in other groups.
• The risk of ectopic pregnancies may be as high as 5 to 6 percent in DES-exposed women, compared with a normal 1 percent.
• There may be an increased risk of prematurity and cervical incompetence in these women as well.

Discouraging as these numbers sound, it is still possible for over 80 percent of DES-exposed women to end up with healthy babies. Anatomical changes in the cervix and uterus, it turns out, do not necessarily mean trouble with pregnancy, although they do signal an increased likelihood for problems.

Women with known DES exposure *in utero* should obtain ob/gyn care from a doctor specializing in this area. Frequent Pap smears are a part of the basic care of these women, and the physician must take time to explain their special needs and listen to their very real concerns. But remember, despite scary statistics, most women exposed to DES *in utero* can expect to achieve a healthy pregnancy and a normal child.

This tragic chapter in the history of obstetrics has taught us to respect the vulnerability of pregnancy even more, and to avoid the use of *all* drugs and chemicals during pregnancy unless they are absolutely proven to be needed, or absolutely proven to be safe. Since absolutes are rare in medicine, caution must be the guiding force.

GYNECOLOGIC PROBLEMS IN PREGNANCY

Women diagnosed during pregnancy with ovarian cysts should be followed closely with pelvic examinations and ultrasound studies. The risk of ovarian cysts being malignant is quite small, but can't be ignored. And noncancerous cysts can cause serious problems (including acute pain and bleeding in the abdomen) if they twist or burst.

Cysts that are seen on ultrasound or are felt during a pelvic exam to be greater than six centimeters (just over two inches) need to be operated upon to rule out cancer. Obviously, burst or twisted cysts will require abdominal surgery as well. In general, a fetus tolerates this type of surgery well, as long as severe peritonitis (abdominal infection) doesn't occur. Anaesthetics used for surgery are, in general, well tolerated in pregnancy; oxygen levels are kept high so the woman and her fetus will be well supplied with this vital element.

Another common gynecologic problem occurring during pregnancy is uterine fibroids—benign muscular growths within the uterus. These will occasionally make conception difficult or may produce miscarriage, depending on their size, type, and location. However, most of the time fibroids cause few problems, despite the fact that the pregnancy hormones will prompt a marked increase in size.

An unusual complication of fibroids during pregnancy is called "degeneration." This process is marked by sometimes severe abdominal pain directly over the fibroid, and is due to the rapid enlargement of the fibroid during the pregnancy. It is treated medically with painkillers (such as Tylenol, Demerol, and codeine) and rest. Degeneration does not usually result in any harm to a woman or to the pregnancy itself. It is rare for fibroids to require surgery during pregnancy.

"Myomectomy" is the name given to the surgical removal of uterine fibroids and reconstruction of the uterus before pregnancy. As many as 40 percent of women who have had this operation for infertility go on to conceive and carry a baby to term. In managing a pregnancy after this operation, the obstetrician will consider the extent of the earlier surgery. If, for example, the endometrial cavity was entered during the operation, or an extensive myomectomy was performed, delivery by cesarean section may be necessary. However, most women who have had myomectomies do not require a c-section and can have a normal vaginal delivery.

PART V

The Infertile Couple

Introduction

In this country today approximately one in ten couples trying to achieve pregnancy is unable to do so. As frightening as that may sound, it is reassuring to know that, for those who do seek medical help, an infertility evaluation can determine the cause of the problem almost 90 percent of the time. And once that happens, at least 60 percent of those previously "infertile" couples can eventually have a baby.

When I say "couple" here, I mean just that. Infertility is a couple's problem: Either or both partners may have conditions that contribute to the inability to conceive. Both partners should seek medical evaluation. Even if only one member of the partnership is discovered to have a physical problem, the problem of infertility itself will still affect both members. This can be a tough circumstance to deal with; infertility and all of the medical evaluations that go along with it can test the very core of a couple's relationship.

From the very start, a gynecologist has several interwoven goals when dealing with infertility:

1. to find the cause of the infertility by means of an orderly, thorough diagnostic work-up
2. to treat the cause of infertility, when feasible, by specific therapy, always trying not to jeopardize the patient's health in another way by doing so

3. to educate both partners in the reproductive process so they can become, through understanding, less anxious about the difficulties they are facing and more involved in any decisions that need to be made
4. to counsel the couples whose infertility therapy is unsuccessful in whatever other options might be available to them.

The number of couples seeking infertility evaluation seems to be increasing every year. This is probably related to delayed childbearing until later in life than used to be common, to the increasing rate of pelvic infections (which can damage the reproductive organs), and to the decreasing number of babies available for adoption. Fortunately, over the past ten years diagnostic methods have also improved, and the ability of gynecologists and fertility specialists to help these couples has increased dramatically.

Fertility rates depend on many things, including age and the frequency of sex. For example, of 100 couples aged eighteen to twenty-eight who have intercourse three or four times a week, about 80 will conceive in one year. The chance during any one cycle is about 15 percent. Half of the 20 percent who did not conceive in a year will achieve conception within a second year. Ten of the original 100 couples, then, will still be unsuccessful after two years. If these 10 couples seek treatment, 5 or 6 will eventually achieve pregnancy.

Professional evaluation of infertility is warranted if there is a failure to conceive after one year of unprotected intercourse. Women over thirty are probably best off seeking fertility evaluation after six months instead of waiting. The reason for this is that the age of the couple—particularly the woman's age—has an impact on infertility rates. It appears that women conceive most easily at about age twenty-four. A slow decline in fertility occurs after thirty, and an accelerated decline begins after thirty-five or forty. The reasons are not entirely known but it has been suggested that ovulation and the production of fertilizable, normal eggs decreases with age. Studies show that conception occurs less frequently with increasing age of the male partner, too.

How often a couple has sex also makes a difference. About four times weekly appears optimal. More frequent sex decreases the number of sperm; less frequent sex lengthens the odds of achieving fertilization. Intercourse must be timed around the anticipated day of ovulation, for the best odds. Other limitations to conception are: 1) the longer the duration of infertility, the less the chances of a successful pregnancy; 2) the more reproductive problems the couple has, the less the chances of success. There is a better chance of success in couples who previously achieved pregnancy but are now unable to do so than in couples who have never achieved pregnancy. It also appears that, when an infertility patient becomes pregnant, there is a slightly higher risk of miscarriage and other problems.

22

The Causes of Infertility

It is obvious that, in order for conception to occur, the woman must ovulate fairly regularly and produce normal eggs, which can move through clear, healthy Fallopian tubes and meet strong, healthy, male sperm at the right time for fertilization. After fertilization the ovum must continue to be transported down the tube into the uterus and be able to burrow into the uterine lining, which must be prepared hormonally to receive it.

Many things may interfere with this normal process. Sometimes a woman or man may have slightly impaired fertility and never know it because the partner has a much higher fertility. But if both partners have fertility that's a bit below normal, that may result in difficulty in conceiving. Sometimes there is no major physical problem; the problem lies simply in lack of knowledge about reproduction—poor sexual technique or incorrect timing of intercourse, for example, or psychological problems in one or both partners or in their interaction that lead to impotence or decreased frequency of sex.

SEXUAL PROBLEMS AND INFERTILITY

Minor physical problems can interfere with satisfactory sex. If the woman has a tight hymen (the piece of tissue around the vaginal opening) it may be painful or impossible for her partner to push his penis completely into her vagina. Incomplete penetration means sperm will not be deposited as close to the cervix as possible, and the discomfort involved may discourage the couple from wanting to have sex at all. Yet this situation can be quickly and easily remedied—often right in the doctor's office—by a small surgical incision in the too-tight hymen.

Sometimes the man is unable to achieve sufficient rigidity of his penis to penetrate his sex partner. Or the woman may involuntarily constrict the muscles of her vagina so that penetration is impossible, a situation called "vaginismus." In either event, the result—unsatisfactory sex—is the same. This may in itself decrease a couple's chances of enjoying sex in the future. Sex therapy can bring about excellent improvement when problems like these exist (see also Chapter 6, "Sexual Function and Dysfunction").

There are certain social and cultural traditions that can interfere with conception. For example, very orthodox Jews do not have sex during menstruation or for one full week after bleeding ceases. If a woman menstruates for eight days and then must wait another seven, ovulation may have already occurred by the time she next has sex.

The infertility work-up itself may prompt sexual difficulties that hamper conception. A couple told to have sex on a regular schedule may immediately lose the desire to have sex at all. What should be a great spontaneous pleasure may now seem mechanical, empty of meaning. Not surprisingly, such feelings may leave a man unable to achieve erection, a woman dry and tight, and both partners unable to reach orgasm. In addition, some specialists feel that stress alone may also affect the ovulatory mechanism so that periods become irregular; and if ovulation does occur the coordinated functioning of the Fallopian tubes may be diminished so the egg and sperm can't be properly transported through them.

THE MALE FACTOR IN INFERTILITY

Only strong, healthy sperm in adequate numbers are capable of producing a pregnancy. A look at a sample of sperm under a microscope (called a "semen analysis") may reveal that a man is producing too few sperm, or that the sperm are not moving vigorously enough to wend their way to an egg, or that the sperm are abnormally shaped.

Male infertility problems may be a result of several types of defect. The structure of some part of the reproductive organs may have been askew from birth, or been damaged by infection, drugs, or accidents. A *varicocele* is an example of a structural problem. This cluster of enlarged veins surrounding the tubes that lead from the testicles to the penis may raise the temperature in this area, resulting in infertility. Even a small varicocele can be associated with infertility. The enlarged veins can be felt if a man's scrotum and testicles are gently examined while he bears down, much as he would during a bowel movement. Varicoceles have been described as feeling like "a bag of worms." The enlarged veins can be removed by surgery.

Another structural problem is a *blockage* in the tubes that sperm pass through on the way from the testes to the penis. In this case, even though sperm are being produced by the testes, they can't get out to fertilize an egg. Some men are born with such a blockage. Others opt for it surgically—in the case of a vasectomy, in which the tubes are severed. The epididymis, a structure through which the sperm pass on their journey from testicle to penis, adds a sperm-nourishing sugar called "fructose" to the semen. If testing the semen reveals no sperm and no "fructose," chances are the problem is an obstruction of the tubes. If, on the other hand, no sperm are present but fructose is detected, then the problem probably lies in an inability of the testicles to manufacture sperm.

Another structural problem leading to male infertility is called "*cryptorchidism.*" In a male fetus the testes are found in the lower abdomen—much like a female's ovaries—but they normally migrate down into the scrotum (the sac of skin behind the penis) by the time a male baby is born. When the testes don't descend into the scrotum the condition that results is cryptorchidism. It severely affects the development of the testes and, if not surgically corrected soon enough, it can prevent normal sperm development entirely. (A baby may also be born without testicles at all. This condition, called "*anorchia,*" obviously results in untreatable sterility.

Another structural abnormality of the male, called "*hypospadias,*" occurs when the opening of the penis is somewhere along the underside of the shaft, back from the tip. This means that at ejaculation sperm are not deposited at the top of the vagina next to the cervix, and the chances of conception are reduced. Pregnancy can often be achieved if a semen sample, collected after masturbation, is deposited next to the cervix, a process called artificial insemination.

Retrograde ejaculation is a condition in which the sperm are pushed backward into the bladder instead of being projected out of the penis at ejaculation. It can be caused by drugs or various types of pelvic surgery, and is diagnosed by finding sperm in the urine instead of in the ejaculate. Infertility from retrograde ejaculation can be treated by threading a tube through the penis into the bladder after ejaculation, and using this sperm sample for artificial insemination.

Infection can also cause male infertility, either temporary or permanent. For example, any significant inflammation of the testes after puberty (as can happen with mumps) may damage the testicles so they can't produce normal sperm. Common infections like gonorrhea, chlamydia, or mycoplasma bacteria have also been implicated in male infertility. Until they are treated with antibiotics these infections can adversely affect both the production of sperm and the fluid portion of semen.

Men can be born with *infertility problems in their genes*. A normal male has 46 chromosomes—22 pairs, plus one X and one Y chromosome that determine his sex. (Normal women also have 46—the same 22 pairs, but with two X's to make them female.) Any variation from this normal chromosome composition often hampers that person's ability to reproduce. In a syndrome called "Kleinfelter's" a man has an extra X—so his cells have 22 chromosome pairs, plus 2 X's and a Y—and is generally unable to father children. Studies done on the chromosomes, then, may be suggested in treating some kinds of male infertility.

Hormonal imbalances in any of the glands of the complex hormone system can cause infertility. A malfunctioning pituitary gland—a kind of master gland that sends signals to other glands throughout the body—can make the testicles poor sperm producers as well as causing thyroid and adrenal gland upsets. A hormonal work-up, which involves checking the levels of various hormones in the blood, is usually done on men with abnormal sperm counts.

Certain drugs and medications can also affect sperm production. Narcotics, alcohol, tranquilizers, some antidepressants, and blood-pressure medications may leave a man unable to ejaculate properly or become erect. Other drugs, such as methotrexate (used to fight cancer and other disorders), antimalaria drugs, nitrofurantoin (an antibiotic), and marijuana, can cause abnormally low sperm production.

And finally, even something as simple as having a job that requires a lot of time sitting—like truck or taxi driving—or wearing tight pants or underwear, can lower a man's sperm count. Since the *testicles are pressed close to the body* for long periods of time, their temperature is raised higher than is optimal for sperm production. Sometimes simply changing from close-fitting jockey shorts to loose, airy boxer shorts which let the testicles fall farther from the body will bring the sperm count back to normal.

Even this partial listing of the types of reproductive problems a man can have should start to make one thing clear: It takes time, patience, determination, and a true "detective's nose" for zeroing in on important clues while not getting bogged down in the mass of potential false leads. And these qualities are called upon from each member of the search party—not only the doctor, but the couple, too.

FEMALE FACTORS IN INFERTILITY

Earlier in this book, I described the complex process of ovulation. As with male fertility problems, things can go awry in almost any step of the way to a woman's pregnancy and cause problems with her fertility.

Hormonal factors can keep a woman's ovaries from releasing an egg (ovulation) or fail to make ready the lining of the uterus to accept an egg once it's fertilized. The most common cause of no ovulation is menopause, when the ovary itself stops working. Although that normally happens when a woman is about fifty to fifty-five years old, premature ovarian failure also occasionally occurs between the ages of thirty and forty, for unknown reasons. Surgical damage to both ovaries and radiation therapy aimed at cancer in the pelvic organs may also produce premature ovarian failure. There is, unfortunately, no treatment that can make the ovaries start up again. However, recent advances in *in vitro* fertilization ("test-tube babies") may make it possible for a woman with nonfunctioning ovaries to carry and deliver a baby. A donor egg, fertilized with her partner's sperm, can be implanted in a woman's uterus and, as long as the uterus itself is healthy, the embryo can develop from then on exactly as her own egg would.

Another type of hormonal problem occurs when the hypothalamus or pituitary areas of the brain fail to signal an egg to develop. Although the ovaries in this case may be perfectly healthy and able to function, ovulation cannot occur without the go-ahead from the brain. Studying the levels of hormones in the blood can uncover the various types of imbalances. Even upsets in glands that have no direct link to the menstrual cycle—like the thyroid, adrenals, and even the pancreas in diabetes—can disturb the body's overall hormonal balance enough to shut down ovulation.

Hormone problems also can prevent a fertilized egg from implanting properly once it reaches the uterus. If not enough progesterone is produced by the ovaries after ovulation, the endometrium will not build up and develop properly. This situation is called "inadequate luteal phase" or "luteal phase defect," since the luteal or after-ovulation half of the cycle is when the problem occurs. Luteal-phase defects can also cause early miscarriage if the endometrium is able to accept implantation of a fertilized egg but then cannot support the growing embryo.

Fallopian tube problems are most likely to be caused by scar tissue. The tubes must be lined with healthy hairlike cilia and be capable of coordinated contractions, so they can move the sperm in one direction, and the egg, before and after fertilization, in the other. The fingerlike projections, called "fimbria," at the end of the tubes must also be able to sweep over the ovary and guide a just-released egg into the tube. Its ability to move freely is an important factor in this process. The inflammation that accompanies infections like gonorrhea and chlamydia can cause scar tissue to form around a tube, in its walls, or inside the channel—leaving it squeezed from without, unable to move properly or blocked off from within. Scar tissue can clump fimbria into a solid immobile mass. Inflammation and infection can also cause a related process, called "adhesion formation," in which tough, thin strands of fibrous tissue, like stringy cobwebs, bind internal organs together. Adhesions can twist the Fallopian tube into such contorted positions that the pickup of an egg is impossible.

Any irritating process in the pelvis—from appendicitis to endometriosis, a condition in which bits of uterine lining stick to pelvic structures instead of being expelled in menstruation—may produce inflammation and scarring in the reproductive organs. The intrauterine (IUD) contraceptive, as previously discussed, can also cause tubal infection and produce tubal scarring, and pelvic surgery or sterilization procedures affect the functioning of the tubes as well.

The role of *the cervix* in conception is to allow sperm to pass through their search for an egg. Vital in this process is the mucus produced by the cervix that fills the canal. Healthy cervical mucus is specially formulated to speed sperm through as quickly and easily as possible. Some women, however, produce too little mucus, while others produce mucus so thick it stops sperm like a barricade. Cervical mucus sometimes contains antibodies which attack and immobilize the sperm as if they were unwanted invaders like bacteria.

The uterus may be unable to accept pregnancy if a woman was born with one of several structural abnormalities. In the most common of these, called a "bicornuate uterus," there is a wall dividing the uterine cavity into two halves, each usually having one Fallopian tube connecting to it. This type of problem can interfere with conception and with the process of pregnancy itself, causing miscarriages and premature delivery.

Another common uterine problem is fibroids. As explained in Chapter 8, "Gynecologic Problems," these noncancerous growths in the walls of the uterus may distort the uterine lining and compress or twist the Fallopian tubes, making implantation or sperm-and-egg travel impossible.

Infertility from No Known Cause

This is one of the most difficult challenges of all. In this small group of infertile couples, all studies are completed and still no reason is found for their inability to conceive. Medical science is simply not advanced enough to completely understand all of the subtle complexities of the process of creating a new human being. As science advances, however, this happens less and less often. We will most likely never know the reasons in every case. Sometimes, however, couples are able to have a child without ever knowing the reason for their previous infertility. As we will see later, extraordinary new treatments, such as *in vitro* fertilization, have started to make this once-impossible dream a reality.

23

Infertility Tests

When a couple goes to a gynecologist or fertility specialist, they usually have two pressing questions: First, why have they been unable to conceive? And, second, what are their chances of being able to have a baby in the future? In spite of their understandable impatience, it usually takes two to six months to be able to completely answer even the first question—why? The success of the treatment and how long it will take depend, of course, on the causes.

Step one of a fertility work-up includes a carefully taken medical history, and a thorough physical examination for both partners. The sperm count is the first basic test for the man. The number, ability to move, and types of sperm in a sample obtained through masturbation are evaluated under a microscope. A count of over 20 million sperm, with 80 percent moving normally and less than 10 percent oddly shaped, is considered normal for one ejaculation. As discussed in the section on causes of male infertility, a genetic work-up and various hormone tests may also be carried out if certain indications exist in the history, physical exam, or sperm count.

For the woman, some basic tests (outlined in Figure 23) are performed during different stages of the menstrual cycle. A "postcoital" test will be performed to see if the cervical mucus is normal. The couple is told to have intercourse at the time ovulation is anticipated. Four to eight hours after intercourse cervical mucus is quickly and painlessly removed from the cervix in the doctor's office for study under the microscope. The number of sperm it contains and their movements will be studied, and the mucus itself will be examined for signs of infection. Poor postcoital test results reveal a low number of sperm,

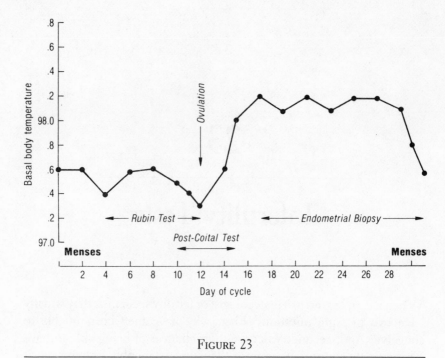

FIGURE 23

Infertility tests and their relationship to the menstrual cycle

and/or sperm that are unable to move correctly. In this case, the cervical mucus may actually be killing the sperm because a cervical infection, hormone imbalance, or immune response has changed its chemical composition.

The health of a woman's uterus may be checked with an "endometrial biopsy" done during the second half of the menstrual cycle. This test involves slipping a narrow instrument through the vagina and cervix and into the uterus, where it snips a tiny chunk of the uterine lining, or endometrium. This tissue may reveal infection, or the endometrium may not have become thick and ready to receive a fertilized egg. The condition called "inadequate luteal phase," due to a deficiency of progesterone, is usually the cause of the second finding.

Another technique discussed earlier, called "hysteroscopy," lets the physician actually see the interior of the uterus, by use of a tiny viewing instrument inserted through the cervix. This technique can reveal a number of abnormalities and irregularities of the endometrium, as well as structural abnormalities of the uterus. A "hysterosalpingogram," in which dye is injected through the cervix and x-rayed as it coats the inside of the uterus and flows out the Fallopian tubes, can spotlight many uterine and tubal abnormalities as well.

The health of the Fallopian tubes can be checked in two additional tests. One, the Rubin or "insufflation" test, is usually done after a menstrual period. Harmless carbon dioxide gas is pumped into the uterus through the cervix. As the gas passes out through the Fallopian tubes into the abdominal cavity, pressure readings are obtained. A fall in pressure means the tubes are open—the gas was able to leak out through them. Your physician may also press a stethoscope to the lower abdomen to listen for the sound of the gas hissing through the tubes. After this test, it is common to experience pain or pressure in one or both shoulders. Although uncomfortable, this "referred pain," due to the gas irritating the diaphragm, is usually a good sign: Its absence would suggest that both tubes were blocked.

The last major test for evaluation of the tubes as well as the pelvic organs in general is "laparoscopy" (see Figure 24). This test most often requires the use of general anaesthesia. Laparoscopy involves pumping carbon dioxide directly into the abdomen, through a small incision made at the edge of the navel, to separate the internal organs enough so individual parts of them can be seen. Next, the laparoscope, the viewing instrument for which the procedure is named, is passed through the incision and into the puffed-up abdominal cavity. The area outside of the tubes, ovaries, and uterus can all be examined. Scar tissue and adhesions may be seen. While the laparoscope is still in place, liquid blue dye is injected through the cervix into the uterus and the doctor waits for it to spill out of the Fallopian tubes—proving they are open. Because laparoscopy can tell a physician so much about the health of the reproductive organs, it is one of the most valuable of all in an infertility investigation. But it is surgery; and it does usually require anaesthesia. So, as small as the risks involved may be—and they *are* small—a physician will not usually opt for a laparoscopy unless easier, quicker, noninvasive tests have proved inconclusive.

The hormone factors that can foul up the process of ovulation also need to be evaluated. A lump of immobile scar tissue blocking a tube is a clear, concrete obstacle to fertility. But the tiny invisible drops of hormones coursing through the blood at the right time and in the right amounts are just as important to the process. For it is these hormones that prompt the body to prepare and release the egg in the first place. Ovulation, as detailed in the chapter on the menstrual cycle, requires

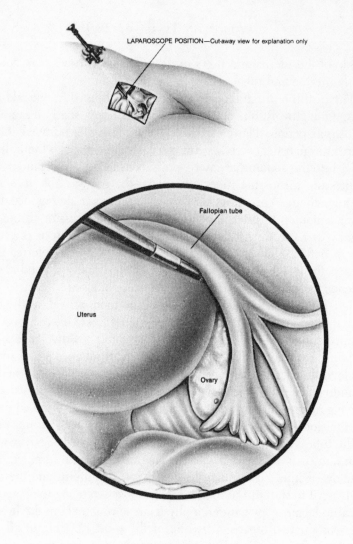

LAPAROSCOPE POSITION—Cut-away view for explanation only

Fallopian tube

Uterus

Ovary

FIGURE 24

Laparoscopy for infertility evaluation

the efficient production of hormones from the pituitary gland, the thyroid gland, and the ovaries themselves. Sometimes these hormones, and others related to the menstrual cycle, can be measured in the blood itself. Measuring FSH, LH, prolactin, thyroid hormone, estrogen, and progesterone levels can confirm that the glands are functioning correctly.

Charting your temperature over a period of one or several months is an indirect way to confirm that ovulation is taking place. A "basal body temperature" (BBT) chart (see Figure 23) is made by taking your temperature every morning as soon as you wake up, before you get out of bed, and drawing a dot on the chart each day at the corresponding temperature. In a normal menstrual cycle, the BBT will show an average low temperature before ovulation with a jump after ovulation. The rise, usually to over 98°, is maintained until menstruation starts. If pregnancy occurs the temperature remains elevated over 98° and, of course, menstruation does not occur. Basal body temperature charting can be used not only to confirm ovulation, but also the existence of a healthy postovulation or luteal phase, as well as an early pregnancy.

Endometrial biopsy, discussed earlier, can also be used to evaluate the functioning of your hormones. In this context, what the physician is searching for is proof that the uterus is responding in synchronization with the menstrual cycle.

Almost all of the tests we've looked at in this chapter are a part of a standard fertility work-up. Although it may seem duplication to do hormone studies—if another test has already shown blocked tubes— it is, in fact, critical that *no one* aspect of a fertility problem be the focus; often there is more than one factor at work, and the second, even third, might be overlooked if the testing were not thorough. It is usually necessary to complete the full work-up and evaluation before embarking on therapy, because therapy depends on exactly what's wrong. A same problem may be treated differently, or not at all, if it is discovered that the woman or the partner has another condition demanding treatment. On average, once a couple has been completely evaluated, it turns out that 40 percent of the time the problems are with the man, 40 percent are with the woman, and 20 percent involve both.

24

The Treatment of Infertility

Once your doctor has the diagnosis of infertility in hand, treatment can begin. As we've said before, it is possible that, in any given couple, more than one cause for infertility may be present and treatment may differ with different combinations of causes. No one wants to plunge into an expensive, complicated treatment regimen only to discover, six months later, that something else entirely was preventing conception. And always the bottom line has to be kept in mind: Successful treatment of infertility is having a baby. Obtaining a normal sperm count, opening blocked Fallopian tubes, making the uterus ready to nourish and support a fertilized egg are all critical parts of the whole; but none of them matters if correcting them doesn't achieve pregnancy.

TREATING MALE INFERTILITY

The two major approaches to the treatment of fertility problems in men are hormone therapy and surgery.

If studies reveal a hormone problem, treatment is usually directed toward replacing what's missing or correcting an imbalance. For example, a thyroid deficiency causing poor sperm production is treated with thyroid hormone to bring the level in the body closer to normal.

Sometimes a man will have a poor sperm count, but his physical and laboratory examinations will have turned up no reason for it. In these cases, testosterone, the male hormone, is sometimes used. In general, unfortunately, it is not very successful. Clomiphene citrate—

a chemical also used to stimulate ovulation in women—has been tried in some hormone imbalances but has not proved promising.

Surgery can be used to repair a varicocele. Each enlarged vein must be tied off individually, in an operation similar to those for hemorrhoids (enlarged veins in the anal canal) and varicose veins (swollen leg veins). The vessels that remain can easily take over the job from the unhealthy ones that are closed off. Varicocele operations can be successful, but it's difficult to know exactly how much help, if any, they will be in any particular man. It is known that the operation is much less effective for men who have sperm counts of under 60 million per ejaculation. But variocele size itself seems to make no difference in how successful the surgery will be. And, to confuse the issue even more, many men with varicoceles have completely normal semen production and sperm counts and no fertility problems at all! The ballpark figure is that 60 percent of the time surgical repair of the varicocele will be a success—one of the more successful forms of therapy in male infertility.

Artificial insemination with the sperm of the male partner may be of some help in cases of low sperm count. This technique involves depositing a man's sperm at the woman's cervix without intercourse. (The sperm is collected by masturbation.) Most often healthy *donor* sperm are used instead of the male partner's poor-quality sperm if both partners agree. (For more on artificial insemination, see later in this chapter.)

TREATING FEMALE INFERTILITY

Failure to ovulate is the most common reproductive problem in women and is, thus, a frequent cause of infertility. A major development of modern gynecology has been production of drugs that can stimulate ovulation. There are two basic types of medication available. One is a man-made chemical—clomiphene citrate. One of its brand names, which may be more familiar, is Clomid. The other is an extract refined from the urine of postmenopausal women and called "pituitary gonadotropin," or "human menopausal gonadotropin" [HMG]. It too has a more familiar brand name: Pergonal.

☐ *Clomiphene citrate: The fertility pill*   is used when a women's ovaries produce estrogen during the first half of the menstrual cycle, but then fail to release an egg or produce progesterone during the second half of the cycle. In about 20 percent of infertile couples, this is the main problem to be overcome. Clomiphene can't help women who do not produce estrogen. Nor is it of use to women who ovulate regularly, except that it is occasionally called in to enhance progesterone production in women with luteal phase defects—women who, in other words, make some progesterone, but not enough.

It's not known exactly how clomiphene works. Somehow it apparently nudges the brain and the pituitary gland, so that the pituitary-released gonadotropins stimulate ovulation.

The drug is given in a start-up dose of 50 milligrams (mg) a day for five days, starting on the fifth day of the menstrual cycle. Ovulation usually occurs within three days after the drug is stopped. If it doesn't, treatment is repeated the next month—and the next if necessary—with a slightly higher dose each time. Each month a careful pelvic examination must be done to see if any cysts have formed on the ovaries or to rule out pregnancy before the next course of treatment is given. Treatment is discontinued for one cycle if ovarian cysts form.

Usually, if the drug is going to work it does so fairly quickly: Most pregnancies occur within the first three cycles. In properly selected patients, 60 percent can be expected to ovulate following clomiphene therapy, and about 40 percent of these become pregnant. In any one cycle, there is a 50/50 chance a pregnancy will occur.

If the drug usually works well, occasionally it works too well. About 8 out of 100 pregnancies will be multiple—mostly twins, with a few cases of triplets or more. Ultrasound can usually reveal the number of eggs that have ripened, and a couple may simply wait until the next cycle to attempt pregnancy if there's evidence of multiple ovulation. Except for the risks involved in a multiple pregnancy (and they are greater than in a single one) clomiphene appears to be very safe for mother and child. There is no increased risk of the baby having a birth defect, and infant survival and performance are normal.

☐ *Pituitary gonadotropin: The fertility shot,* which is also called "human menopausal gonadotropin" [HMG], or Pergonal, is expensive. Treatment, which involves daily injections for approximately nine days, may cost over $500 per cycle. Fortunately, it is also effective. Almost 90 percent of women with ovaries capable of responding will do so after the following treatment schedule: Most patients will be ready to ovulate after being given two ampules of HMG per day for seven to twelve days. Unlike clomiphene, which stimulates the ovaries via the brain, HMG works directly on the ovaries. The amount of estrogen the ovaries are producing is carefully monitored with frequent blood tests. Then, when critical levels are achieved, and the follicle of the ovary has matured, a second drug, human chorionic gonadotropin or HCG, is injected to prompt actual release of the egg—ovulation.

The pregnancy rate with this method is approximately 50 to 75 percent. There is no evidence of an increased risk of birth defects in babies born to mothers who have undergone this treatment regimen; but here again, there is a risk of multiple pregnancy—as much as one in five (20 percent). Fifteen percent are twins and 5 percent of the pregnancies that result are of three or more. (Of course, since such multiple pregnancies are due to multiple ovulation, the siblings are not identical.) In multiple pregnancies there is a higher chance of both prematurity and miscarriage. The miscarriage rate is, in fact, approximately 20 percent.

☐ *Hyperprolactinemia*, a problem with the area of the brain's "master gland," the pituitary, which causes too much of the hormone prolactin to be produced, has recently been identified. One theory is that tiny, microscopic tumors in this area of the brain might be to blame. Normally, prolactin is involved with milk production after birth. At that time it appears also to be involved with suppressing ovulation—possibly as a kind of built-in birth control that prevents, although not infallibly, a new pregnancy from starting too soon after the last has ended. Likewise, the excess hormonal secretion interferes with ovulation, even if it happens when a woman is not nursing.

Treatment for so-called hyperprolactinemia, which can be detected by a blood test, involves the use of the drug bromocriptine mesylate. This drug curbs the production of prolactin by the pituitary and shrinks the microtumors. The measurement of prolactin is one of the basic tests in the hormonal evaluation of infertility.

☐ *Treating the cervix* for abnormalities can be attempted with several procedures: special douches that enhance sperm migration, small doses of estrogens that improve cervical mucus, antibiotics (either in pills to take by mouth or suppositories to insert vaginally) to treat infections, or with cryotherapy to literally quick-freeze abnormal tissue. Although abnormal antibodies can be detected with special test techniques, a successful way to treat this problem has not yet been discovered.

☐ *Treating uterine problems* depends on the nature of the problem. If, for example, the endometrium does not become ready for implantation each month, the problem is generally a hormonal one, and may be treated by ovulation-induction techniques.

Fibroids may require an operation called "myomectomy." This involves surgically removing the tumors from within the muscle mass of the uterine walls. If the fibroids are actually responsible for infertility in a particular case (difficult to determine for sure), this type of surgery can be quite successful. Some congenital abnormalities, such as a bicornuate uterus, can also be treated with surgery, if necessary. An abnormally shaped uterus isn't actually considered to be a common cause of female infertility, however. When it does cause problems they will more often be repeated miscarriages or prematurity. Most often a woman born with an unusually shaped uterus will have no problems bearing children at all.

☐ *Treating tube problems* may involve any of many surgical techniques that reopen blocked Fallopian tubes or cut away scar tissue that's choking them from the outside. Even if that works, however, the true success rate is not great: In the most experienced hands pregnancy is achieved only about half the time. The Fallopian tubes are extremely delicate structures, and despite meticulous, extraordinarily precise microsurgical techniques, normal egg and sperm movement through them may not occur.

Tubal surgery is also known to increase the risk of ectopic pregnancy (a pregnancy occurring in the tube itself). This happens only once or twice for every 100 pregnancies in the general population, but happens in an extremely high 15 to 20 per 100 pregnancies following tubal surgery. Any woman who has undergone tubal surgery and subsequently becomes pregnant must have an ectopic pregnancy ruled out as early as possible. If allowed to continue, such a pregnancy can rupture the tube, causing serious internal bleeding and even death. Fortunately this situation can be discovered more quickly today than ever before by careful measurement of chorionic gonadotropin and with early use of ultrasound.

Before undergoing tubal surgery, the couple—the woman in particular—must understand the risks of the procedure, the likelihood of success, and what alternatives there may be. Some of the optimism about and enthusiasm for tubal surgery has recently abated since the success rates of *in vitro* fertilization have improved. In some cases, *in vitro* simply bypasses closed tubes and allows for pregnancy.

The Latest Approaches to Treating Infertility

☐ *In vitro fertilization:* "Test tube" babies are the successful result of bypassing malfunctioning Fallopian tubes. *In vitro* fertilization (IVF) is, basically, the attempt to solve the problem of blocked or damaged Fallopian tubes by simply leapfrogging their role altogether. This process was first successful with the birth of Louise Brown in 1978, through the work of two Englishmen, Dr. Patrick Steptoe and Robert Edwards. The National Academy of Sciences estimated that between one in 200 and one in 100 of all American women who are otherwise unable to bear children might be able to do so through IVF.

The process consists of four basic steps. The egg must be removed from a woman's ovaries, fertilized, allowed to grow a determined amount in a "test tube" (usually, actually a flat, round dish), and then put back into the woman's uterus to implant. From then on the pregnancy is exactly like any other. The first two steps are relatively simple. Obtaining the ovum and fertilization are usually successful. The harder part comes later. Most unsuccessful attempts at IVF are due to the inability of the embryo to implant in the uterine lining. And in IVF the general rule of successful infertility treatment remains the same: Half-measures don't count; the success rate is the number of births.

In a woman's body, there is only a short period—about three hours—when eggs are fully mature and ripe for fertilization. The woman's cycle, then, must be monitored extremely carefully in order to remove the egg at precisely the right time. The drugs clomiphene (Clomid) and human menopausal gonadotropin (Pergonal) are used here to stimulate the production of eggs, just as they are for women whose ovaries are not ovulating spontaneously. Very often these drugs cause more than one egg to develop. But now what is usually a drawback—the risk of multiple births—is a plus. It increases the chances of an IVF success. In fact, on the average, 5.3 eggs can be obtained per woman. By obtaining multiple eggs, the chances of fertilizing one that will successfully "take" are increased. Usually, up to three fertilized eggs are replaced.

The procedure used in most IVF clinics is fairly standard. Typically, a woman receives Pergonal three days after menstruation begins in

TABLE 10

METHODS OF PROCREATION

CODE

$\frac{♀}{M}$	Mother's ovum	$\frac{♂}{D}$	Donor's sperm
$\frac{♀}{D}$	Donor's ovum	$\frac{☺}{M}$	Child borne by mother
$\frac{♂}{F}$	Father's sperm	$\frac{☺}{SM}$	Child borne by surrogate mother

+ Natural fertilization   ⊕ *In vitro* fertilization   A+ Artificial fertilization

= No transfer of embryo   ⊖ Embryo transfer

PROBLEM	SOLUTION					
Normal (no problem)	$\frac{♀}{M}$	+	$\frac{♂}{F}$	=	$\frac{☺}{M}$	
Father infertile (no sperm)	$\frac{♀}{M}$	A+	$\frac{♂}{D}$	=	$\frac{☺}{M}$	
Father infertile Mother fertile but unable to carry pregnancy (no sperm & closed tubes)	$\frac{♀}{M}$	⊕	$\frac{♂}{D}$	=	$\frac{☺}{M}$	
Father infertile Mother fertile but unable to carry pregnancy (no sperm or uterus)	$\frac{♀}{M}$	⊕	$\frac{♂}{D}$	=	$\frac{☺}{SM}$	
Father infertile Mother infertile, able to carry pregnancy (no sperm & no ovarian function)	$\frac{♀}{D}$ $\frac{♀}{D}$	A+ +	$\frac{♂}{D}$ $\frac{♂}{D}$	⊖ ⊖	$\frac{☺}{M}$ $\frac{☺}{M}$	or
Father fertile Mother infertile and unable to carry pregnancy (no ovaries or uterus)	$\frac{♀}{D}$	A+	$\frac{♂}{F}$	=	$\frac{☺}{SM}$	

PROBLEM	SOLUTION				
Father fertile	♀	A+	♂	⊖	☺
Mother infertile	D		F		M or
and able to carry pregnancy	♀	⊕	♂		
(no ovarian function)	D		F	=	☺
					M
Father fertile	♀	⊕	♂	=	☺
Mother fertile	M		F		M
but unable to conceive					
Father fertile	♀	⊕	♂	⊖	☺
Mother fertile	M		F		SM
but cannot carry pregnancy					
(no uterus)					
Father infertile	♀	+	♂	=	☺
Mother infertile	D		D		SM
and unable to carry pregnancy					
(adoption)					

order to stimulate her ovaries to mature several eggs during the next cycle. The approach of ovulation must be monitored extremely closely so the short hours of prime readiness are not missed. Blood tests check for rising estrogen levels; ultrasound scans of the ovary measure the size of the follicles, the tiny sacs in which the eggs mature. After two weeks the follicles should be close to the right size, and the woman is given a shot of HCG, which will bring on ovulation within thirty-eight hours.

Just before ovulation occurs, the egg is carefully removed, a process which requires anaesthesia. The surgeon makes a tiny incision in the woman's abdomen, then threads a thin hollow needle toward the ovary. A laparoscope (discussed earlier) is used to help guide the needle, which pierces the follicle (or follicles, one at a time) and gently sucks out the fluid in it. The follicular fluid is then rushed to an adjoining laboratory and checked under a microscope to make sure that at least one egg has been retrieved. Recently, ultrasound has been used experimentally to guide a needle to the follicles by way of the vagina. This technique, if successful, will eliminate the need for the laparoscope and anaesthesia.

The ova are carefully washed and placed in small, round petri dishes that contain a mixture of nutrients designed to help the eggs grow. These petri dishes are incubated for four to eight hours at body temperature. Meanwhile, sperm which have been spun out of their semen with a centrifuge are washed and incubated in their own dish. After incubation, 500,000 to 1.5 million sperm are transferred into each egg-bearing petri dish. Sometime during the next twenty-four hours, if all goes well, fertilization will occur.

Just a few hours after fertilization, the zygote (or fertilized egg) is put into a new solution—this one specially formulated to support cell division and the maturing of the embryo. This is a critical time if development is to proceed normally. A proper balance of nutrients, carefully monitored temperature, and a good supply of oxygen are all essential. Even so, only a small percentage of embryos will develop through the blastocyst stage—the point at which the embryo has sixteen cells. And sixteen cells is IVF's magic number: The embryo is ready for implantation.

Of course, these carefully nurtured embryos can't just be plunked back into the uterus at any time. As much as can be judged, implantation must be timed so that the endometrium is exactly at the right stage to accept the embryo. Unfortunately, at the current stage of medical knowledge, there is simply no way to be sure that the "test tube" embryo has developed at precisely the same speed as it would have in the body. A discrepancy between the readiness of the uterus and that of the egg is believed to be largely responsible for failed *in vitro* attempts.

Actually depositing the tiny, growing embryo into the uterus requires no anaesthetic, but it demands a skilled physician. The uterus does not like things being put into it and responds to such attempts by contracting to push them out. The embryos must be carefully drawn up into a narrow Teflon tube, then slid through the cervix and into the uterus with as little disturbance as possible.

Now the embryo (or embryos—many clinics will transfer more than one at a time to better the chances of pregnancy) is on its own. Although the woman takes progesterone to keep the lining of her uterus receptive, there is nothing more that science can do at this point to encourage the embryo to burrow into the endometrium and grow. All that can be done is to watch and wait. Periodic samples of the woman's blood will be taken to check whether HCG levels are going up—a sign of pregnancy.

There is little more than a 20 percent—one in five—chance of a successful pregnancy even in the most experienced hands. Even once implantation occurs, as many as one-third of IVF pregnancies spontaneously miscarry in the first three months. But while this is, clearly, a much higher than normal rate, a few important points must be kept in mind. For one thing, many of the protective mechanisms of *in vivo* (in the body) fertilization do not exist in the glass dishes of a lab. Normally, cervical mucus and the area where the tubes meet the uterus act as filtering stations, to keep abnormal sperm from getting through. Also, since there is a much greater number of sperm exposed to an egg in the dishes, there is a higher chance of an abnormal fertilization by more than one sperm. Embryos such as these will be spontaneously aborted. It's the body's backup screening to eliminate—early and easily—embryos that could not possibly survive anyway. It is also possible that the various stages of the procedure, including drug treatment and laparoscopy, may damage the lining of the uterus, leading to some of the early miscarriages. As more and more experience is gained in *in vitro* fertilization, perhaps these numbers will go down.

In vitro fertilization has primarily focused on infertile women with blocked Fallopian tubes. Occasionally, though, it has been used to bypass a blockage of the vas deferens—the narrow tubes sperm take from testicles to penis. If—through a small incision—the sperm can be removed from the testes before the block in the vas deferens, they may then be used to fertilize an egg by the *in vitro* method. (*In vitro* is more efficient in this case than artificial insemination since there are fewer sperm.)

☐ *Artificial insemination and embryo transfer* is another science-engineered way to beat fertility problems of a different sort. This method involves depositing semen, via a syringe, right at a woman's cervix. In this country, an estimated 10,000 conceptions a year are due to this very successful method. There are two types of artificial insemination (AI). When the semen is obtained from a woman's partner, it's called "homologous" artificial insemination (HAI). "Heterologous" is the term used when the semen is from a donor. To avoid confusion, the latter is usually dubbed "AID"—for "artificial insemination by donor." All donors are screened for genetic defects, infections, acquired immune deficiency syndrome, and fertility potential before their semen is accepted.

HAI may be done if physical or psychological problems prevent a couple from being able to achieve fertilization through intercourse. For example, the sperm from several ejaculates can be pooled and deposited near the cervix in concentrated form to compensate for poor sperm production. Another method is called the "split ejaculate." Since the first part of the ejaculate tends to contain the most active and well-developed sperm, this portion is separated from the less potent second part for insemination.

Artificial insemination by donor may be indicated if the partner is sterile—that is, producing no sperm—or when there is a risk of passing along a hereditary disease in the partner's genes. Artificial insemination is also used when there is severe Rh incompatibility (as explained in Chapter 21) and in most cases of deficient sperm production. AID also allows women without partners to bear children.

The availability of a method known as "cryopreservation" has broadened the potential for artificial insemination. Cryopreservation is a technique of freezing and preserving of sperm by immersing tubes of semen in liquid nitrogen that's kept at 320° below zero. At these temperatures the sperm may be stored for years. "Cryobanks" make it possible for a man to store his semen before undergoing a vasectomy— in case he should one day in the future wish to have a child.

Cryopreservation is also being tested for use with in vitro fertilization. Several embryos may be frozen in liquid nitrogen, then thawed and inserted if the initial embryo does not implant or miscarries. Although this eliminates the need to repeat the process of egg retrieval and fertilization, 30 to 50 percent of embryos do not survive the deep freeze. If they make it, however, thawed embryos have a higher chance of implanting since the woman has not been given extra hormones to stimulate ovulation as is done to retrieve eggs. Therefore the cycle is a more natural and normal one, and the endometrium is healthy.

Sperm isn't the only reproductive product that can be donated. Eggs may be donated as well. Fertilization of a donor egg by either a male donor's sperm or the partner's sperm may be done in a petri dish, much like standard in vitro techniques. The only difference is that the embryo is put into an infertile woman's uterus, rather than the female donor's.

Fertilization of a donor egg may also occur in the donor's own body in a relatively new procedure known as "embryo transfer." In this method, a fertile woman (the donor) is artificially inseminated with semen from an infertile woman's partner. Five days after fertilization the embryo is flushed out of the donor's uterus with a nutrient solution and then implanted in the infertile woman's uterus. This painless procedure is called "lavage," which means "washing."

There are advantages and disadvantages to embryo transfer. Embryo transfer theoretically enables doctors to extend the childbearing years of women past menopause. It may also allow women whose infertility is caused by malfunctioning ovaries as well as blocked Fallopian tubes to experience pregnancy. Women who might pass on an inheritable disease are able to bear children without that risk. (Egg donors, like sperm donors, are carefully screened.) However, there is a risk that flushing may not recover an embryo from the donor's uterus; and she could be left with an unwanted pregnancy. Because of these unanswered questions, this technique is still considered to be experimental.

□ *Surrogate Motherhood* is the use of another new, controversial method of reproduction: A fertile woman may be hired by an infertile couple to bear their child. This is illegal in some states because it is considered sale of an infant, while other states allow it. A surrogate mother may be artificially inseminated with the partner's sperm. Or, in cases in which the woman's ovaries can produce a normal egg but her uterus is not able to carry the child, the surrogate mother may be the recipient of an embryo which has been fertilized either in the other woman's uterus or in a petri dish. The surrogate mother then carries the fetus to full term and, upon delivery, relinquishes the baby to the couple. In theory it is simple, but in fact legal problems may arise.

Moral and ethical questions are inevitable with *in vitro* fertilization, artificial insemination, embryo transfer, and surrogate motherhood, stemming from the fact that some of the natural steps in the process of reproduction are being replaced by artificial methods. Artificial insemination bypasses sexual intercourse, while *in vitro* fertilization not only does that but replaces tubal fertilization with fertilization in a dish in a lab. Many of the arguments concerning these reproductive technologies are similar to the ethical arguments over other "unnatural" life support aids, like the artificial heart. These are issues a couple should consider, together with their doctor and maybe their pastor, rabbi, or even lawyer before making a decision.

The possibilities for procreation with the use of *in vitro* fertilization and artificial insemination are vast (see Table 10). The methods themselves are often time-consuming, extremely costly, psychologically challenging. The moral questions raised may be difficult to wrestle with. And in most cases, the legality of these possibilities has yet to be considered. But modern medicine is now able to give children to some couples who would otherwise be childless. To an infertile couple yearning for a family, that possibility may make all the struggles worthwhile.

Conclusion

I have worked in the field of reproductive health for over twenty years now. During that time almost every aspect of obstetrics has benefited from tremendous advances in medical knowledge. Many of the medical discoveries that were discussed in this book simply didn't exist two decades ago: the now widely available procedure of amniocentesis that lets us check on the health of the unborn fetus; the advanced fertility tests with which we can pinpoint many problems of conception; the still-developing techniques of *in vitro* fertilization that allow previously infertile couples to achieve pregnancy; and the sophisticated monitors that alert us to the early signs of distress in a baby during delivery. Countless couples have healthy babies today because of these, and other, technological wonders.

But it's not only high-tech machines and sophisticated procedures that have brought the miraculous process of having a baby out of the dark ages and into the forefront of science. We have learned so much more about the intricate functioning of the human body: subtle details of how the organs of reproduction work; how a fetus is first conceived and then develops; how the complex interrelationship between mother and fetus is maintained. And we have learned so much more about the tremendous impact seemingly minor things can have on a woman's overall health and fertility—eating correctly during pregnancy, for example, and avoiding cigarettes, alcohol, and all but doctor-approved drugs.

What is important and striking about these findings is that women have so much control over most of them. So while technology has given health professionals new tools that have bettered each woman's odds of bearing a healthy baby, increased knowledge has given women, too, a new measure of responsibility for their pregnancies. Today, women and their doctors find themselves working as a team to ensure that a pregnancy proceeds as smoothly and healthily as possible.

Now that we've come so far, we have the challenge and the opportunity to take reproductive health even further, to start thinking about reproductive health as a lifestyle that starts not with conception but long before. That is what this book is all about. The earlier you start taking care of your body, the better your chances of being able to conceive and bear a healthy child when the time comes. It can make a difference that, ten years before conception, you went straight to your doctor at the first sign of a vaginal infection. Your choice of birth control was, and is, important. How you're eating and exercising today may make a difference. And so much more. Our goal is to achieve healthier pregnancies—during which a woman will feel happy and healthy and be able to handle most of the same activities she has always handled. And, finally, our goal is healthier babies who come into the world with the best possible chance for a long, productive life.

Index

Abdomen, 30, 59, 75–76, 79, 93, 98, 136, 140, 174–75, 181, 191, 196, 199, 203, 205, 210–11, 219, 221, 223, 232, 239, 249

Abnormalities, 50, 84, 115, 120, 131, 144, 147, 150, 155, 192–193, 196, 202, 204, 208–9, 213, 238–39, 245–46

Abortion, xi, xvii, 41–42, 50, 52, 84, 112, 148, 153, 195, 210: complete, 193; missed, 192–93; spontaneous, 119, 138, 143, 145, 173, 186, 190–93, 195, 209, 214–16, 222; threatened, 194

Abscess, Bartholin, 80–81

Abstinence, from drinking, 145; sexual, 54

Acetylcholinesterase, 201, 202

Acid base balance (pH), 35, 211

Acne, 48

Acquired immune deficiency syndrome. See AIDS

Acyclovir, 77

Adhesions, 97 (fig. 14), 235, 239

Adrenal gland, 233–34

Aerobic exercise, 27, 30–31, 131–32, 138

AFP. See Alpha–fetoprotein test

Age, maternal, 117–21

AI. See Insemination, artificial

AID. See Heterologous artificial insemination

AIDS, 86–87, 251

AIDS–Related Complex (ARC), 87

Alkylating agents, 144

Allergies, 17, 57, 83, 85

Alpha-fetoprotein test. See Tests

Amenorrhea, 13–14: definition of, 13

American Association of Sex Educators, Counselors and Therapists, 70

American Board of Obstetrics and Gynecology, 55, 172–73

American Cancer Society, 22, 24, 99

American College of Nurse Midwives, 173

American College of Obstetricians and Gynecologists (ACOG), 56, 134–38, 173, 176, 177

Amino acids, 34–35, 37, 125

Amniocentesis, xiv, xvii, 108, 152, 154, 161, 167, 201, 202, 205, 207 (fig. 22), 208–9, 215, 216, 255

Amniotic fluid, xiv, 123, 124 (fig. 15), 149, 166, 167, 201–2, 207 (fig. 22), 208: sac, 78, 114, 146, 166, 175–76, 192, 204–5, 210

Amphetamines. See Drugs

123, 135, 173–74: drop in, 179; high, xii–xiii, 29, 57, 137, 161, 200, 213, 218; medications, 233
Bonding, 205
Bone, 25–26, 36, 96, 126, 149, 171, 174–75, 183–84, 191, 201, 203–4
Bow type of IUD, 51
Bowels, 72, 89–90, 98, 180: disease, xvii, 96, 219; movements, 59, 79–80, 90, 97, 127, 175, 180, 232
Bra, support, 140, 179
Brain, 29, 38, 84, 152, 200–201, 234, 244–45: embryonic, 166, 199
Braxton Hicks contractions, 175, 178–79
Breakthrough bleeding, 49
Breast, 3, 18–24, 47–48, 55, 57, 123, 124 (fig. 15), 140, 157, 174, 178–79, 183, 220–22: operation, 184. *See also* Areola; Cancer; Dimpling; Lumps; Mammography; Nipples; Self-examination; Trauma
Breastfeeding, 11, 18–19, 23, 35, 78, 90, 123, 127, 189, 221–22, 245
Breath, shortness of, 30, 50, 118, 180
Breathing, 32, 37–38, 140: exercises, 187; fetal, 166–67, 204; of newborn, 208
Bromocriptine mesylate, 245
Brown, Louise, 247
BSU pregnancy blood test. *See* Tests
Burning (symptom), 71, 73–74, 76–77, 79, 83, 181

Caffeine, 145–46
Calcium, 25, 36, 123, 125–26, 179, 182
Calories, 26–27, 33–34, 37–39, 122–24, 127–28, 129, 136, 140
Cancer, 18, 22–24, 33, 44, 47–48, 52–53, 55, 59–60, 67, 77–78, 92, 98, 103, 115, 142, 144, 174, 200, 222–23, 233–34. See also *Carcinoma in situ*
Candeptin, 72
Candida albicans, 71
Carbohydrates, 32–33, 36, 39, 124, 127, 129

Carcinoma in situ, 98, 100, 102–3
Cardiac: reserve, 138–39; output, 131
Cardiovascular efficiency, 26, 31
Cardiovascular system, 131, 137
Career, xi–xii, 40, 88, 108, 110–13
Carriers, 151–54, 217
Cells, 148–51, 154, 250; blood cells, 11, 25, 79, 125, 132, 149–50, 174, 208, 214–15
Cereal, 35, 127, 180
Cervical caps, 41, 44–45
Cervicitis, 74
Cervix, 5, 7, 8 (fig. 4), 15, 42–45, 47, 52, 54, 58–59, 66–67, 74, 76, 81, 83, 86, 90, 92, 100–101, 164, 174–76, 209, 211, 216n, 223, 230, 232, 235, 237–239, 243, 245, 250–52: incompetent, 102, 138, 184, 192, 194–195, 222; opening (dilatation) of, 179, 193; thinning (effacement) of, 179
Cesarean section, 78, 94, 119, 188, 200, 208, 211, 213, 217, 224
Chancre, 84
Chancroid, 85
Checkups, 56–57, 91, 116
Cheese, 35, 126–27, 140
Chemicals, 116, 141–46, 153, 156, 193, 223, 243
Chemotherapy, 221
Cherry, S. H., 38, 189
Child-rearing, 137, 161
Childbearing, xvii, 51, 102, 117, 131, 154, 161, 198, 224, 228, 242, 246, 248–49, 252, 256: years, 88, 91, 95, 220, 222, 253
Childbirth, xvii, 7, 42, 55, 94, 109, 113–14, 134, 170, 187–89, 191, 194–95, 205, 211, 212, 215, 221, 245, 247. *See also* Delivery
Children, 110–11, 113, 142, 144, 147, 199, 218: born to AIDS–infected mothers, 86; care of, 12; female, 56; with genetic problems, 153
Chlamydia, 74, 81–82, 99, 193, 195, 233, 235
Chloasma (liver spots), 48–49
Chloramphenicol, 144
Cholesterol, 28, 219
Chorion, 209

28–29; low-density (LDL), 28–29
Lippe's Loop, 51
Lithium, 144
Liver: as food, 127; in body, 200
Lobules, definition of, 18
Loopy type of IUD, 5
LSD. See Drugs
Lubrication, vaginal, 64, 66, 80
Lumps, in breasts, 179
Lungs, xvii, 49, 180, 208, 215, 217
Luteal phase, 241: inadequate, 192, 235, 238, 244
Lymphatic systems, 37, 77, 85, 103
Lymphogranuloma venereum (LGV), 85

Macronutrients, 36
Magnesium, 36
Male reproductive organs, 231–34
Malformations, 144, 146, 193, 216: congenital, xiv, 147, 150, 220. See also Limbs; Uterus
Mammography, 21–22, 24
March of Dimes Program, 148
Marijuana. See Drugs
Marriage, 185: early, 99; late, xii
Marsupialization, 81
Masters and Johnson, 67–68
Mastitis, 22
Masturbation, 65, 69, 232, 237, 243
Maternity: benefits, 112, 115–16
Mattress, firm, 180
Meat, 34–35, 124–25, 140, 158
Medications, xii, 67, 72, 74, 107, 141–46, 158, 181–82, 187, 214, 217–18, 233, 243
Men: bisexual, 86–87; circumcised, 99; fertility problems in, 222; heterosexual, 86; older, 65, 169, 228; uncircumcised, 73, 99. See also Homosexual men
Mendel, Gregor, 151
Mendelian (single gene) disorders, 148, 151–53, 155
Menopause, 10, 13–14, 21–23, 55, 91–94, 118, 234, 253
Menstruation, 3, 7, 9, 17, 21–23, 44, 47, 55, 57, 72, 88–90, 93–95, 97–98, 102, 231, 235: cycle, 9–15, 17, 19, 48–49, 53–54, 77, 89–93, 95, 118–19, 121,

163–65, 169, 171, 195, 228, 234, 237, 238 (fig. 23), 239–40, 243–44, 247; flow, 13–15, 48, 53, 72, 90–92, 143, 164. See also Periods
Mental: health, 25, 31; retardation, xvii, 143, 150, 152
Mercury, 115
Metabolism, 26–27, 34, 37–38, 125, 140, 147, 152, 165, 179, 213
Methotrexate, 233
Metronidazole (Flagyl), 73
Micronutrients, 36
Midwife, 172–73
Migraine headaches, 47
Milk, 34–35, 124–27, 182
Milk-production, 18–19, 127, 129, 221–22, 245: glands, 179
Minerals, 32–33, 35–37, 115, 124–125
Miscarriage, xvi, xvii, 48, 52, 92, 94, 113, 115–16, 119–20, 142–43, 145–46, 148, 161, 169, 173, 175, 186, 190–96, 200, 207, 209, 214–15, 222–23, 229, 235–36, 245–46, 251: incomplete, 193; multiple, 195
Mittelschmerz, 97
Monistat, 72
Mons veneris, 5
Mood changes, 49, 178, 185
Moral questions, 253–54
Morning sickness, 182
Morning-after pill, 50
Mucus, 5–6, 15–16, 47, 80, 164, 235, 237–38, 245, 251: membranes, 182
Multifactorial disorders, 148, 153
Mumps, 177, 233
Muscles, 7, 26–28, 30, 36, 65, 84, 96, 117, 127, 135–37, 139–40, 144, 164, 179, 231, 246: fetal, 204
Muscular dystrophy, 153
Mutations, 151
Mycoplasma, 193, 195, 233
Mycostatin, 72
Myomectomy, 94, 224, 246

Nails, fetal, 166, 167
Naps, 181. See also Sleep
Narcotics, 144, 233. See also Drugs

National Academy of Sciences, 247
National Foundation for Ileitis and
    Colitis, 219
National Genetics Foundation, 155
Nausea, 48, 50, 73, 114, 176, 182,
    185. *See also* Morning sickness
Navel, 167, 239
Needles, 87, 203, 205, 249
Neonatology, xiv. *See also* Newborn
Nerves, 5–7, 36, 67, 75–76, 179
Nervous system, 152–53, 200–203
Neural tube defect, 200–201, 202–
    203
Neurologists, 153
Newborn, 78, 83, 189, 217
Nickel, 36
Nipples, 18–20, 179, 183
Nitrofurantoin, 233
Nodules, 23
Nonoxynol–9, 45
Nose: embryonic, 166; stuffy, 178,
    182
Nursing. *See* Breastfeeding
Nutrition, xvii, 3, 10, 32–39, 56,
    122–29, 133, 146, 156–57

Obesity, 123, 138, 200, 213–14. *See
    also* Overweight problems
Obstetricians, passim.
Odors, 15–16, 72–74
Orgasm, 7, 54, 64–66, 68–69, 231
Ovarian: masses, 204; pregnancy, 196
Ovaries, 8 (figs. 4, 5), 12, 14, 18, 23,
    59, 66, 74, 89 (fig. 11), 90–91,
    94, 95 (fig. 13), 96, 97 (fig. 14),
    102, 118, 150 (fig. 17), 163,
    232, 234–35, 239, 240 (fig. 24),
    243–45, 247–49, 253
Overheating, 139
Overweight problems, xvii, 26, 130–
    131, 213–14
Ovulation, 10, 12–13, 16, 46–49, 53
    (fig. 8), 54, 64, 97, 118, 163–
    164, 165 (fig. 18), 167, 168, 171,
    213–14, 228, 230–31, 234–35,
    237, 238 (fig. 23), 239–41, 243–
    247, 249, 252
Ovum, 52, 148, 150 (fig. 17), 163–
    164, 230, 247–48, 250–51:
    blighted, 192; donor's, 248. *See
    also* Eggs
Oxygen, 26, 28–30, 36, 38, 130,

132, 146, 174, 184, 208, 223,
    250

Pain, 21, 47, 49, 67, 75–76, 83, 90,
    97–98, 100, 140, 175, 179, 184,
    187, 191, 193, 196, 203, 205,
    223
Pap smear (Pap test), 47, 58 (fig. 9),
    59, 77, 98–103, 157, 174, 221
Papanicolaou, George N., 58, 100
Papilloma virus, 78
Pasta, 181–82
Pediatrician, 56, 111
Pelvic inflammatory disease (PID),
    52, 74, 82–83, 96–97 (fig. 14)
Pelvic tilt, 136–37
Pelvis, 5–17, 42, 64–67, 74, 91, 96–
    98, 136–37, 157, 171, 174–75,
    197, 221, 228, 235
Penicillin, 83, 85
Penis, 5–6, 46, 54, 79, 81–82, 84–
    85, 99, 230–32, 251
Pergonal, 244
Perinatology, xiv, 173, 205, 208
Perineum, 8 (fig. 5): definition of, 5
Periods (of menstruation), 3, 13–14,
    17, 19, 49, 52, 90–92, 97, 118,
    121, 142, 158, 163–68, 170–71,
    173, 182, 191, 194, 196, 231,
    239: painful (dysmenorrhea), 90
Pesticides, 141
pH. *See* Acid base balance
Phenobarbital, 220
Phenylketonuria (PKU), 152
Phosphorus, 182
Photographs of fetus, 204–5, 206
Physical activity, 122, 136, 196
Pill, fertility, 243–44
Pills for birth control, 15, 41–42,
    46–51, 71–72, 87, 90–91, 157,
    169: side effects, 47–50, 183.
    See also Morning-after pill
Pituitary: gland of the brain, 10–11,
    233–34, 240, 244–45; gonado-
    tropin, 243–45
PKU. *See* Phenylketonuria
Placenta, 123, 124 (fig. 15), 131–32,
    140, 165–67, 203–5, 207 (fig.
    22), 209–10, 214–15, 217–19:
    previa, 138
Plaques in blood, 28–29
Plateau phase, 64–65

Vasectomy, 232, 252
VDRL test, 84
Vegetables, 33–35, 126–27
Vegetarian diet, 32, 35, 124: lacto-ovo, 125
Veins, 37, 49, 136, 179–81, 232, 243: varicose, 180–81, 243. *See also* Vena cava; Variocele
Vena cava, 136, 140
Venereal disease (VD), 81–82, 173
Venereal Disease Research Laboratory, 84
Videotape of exercises, 134
Virus, 75–78, 86–87, 176, 200, 216–17, 222
Vision, blurred, 50, 175
Vitamins, 32–33, 35–37, 123–25, 127, 174, 194
Vomiting, 37, 50, 114, 176, 182, 185. *See also* Morning sickness
Vulva, 72, 75, 78, 85

Walking, 27–31, 38, 133–35, 139, 180
Warm-up, 31, 135, 139
Warts, 183: genital (condyloma accuminata), 78, 99. *See also* Papilloma virus
Wassermann, August P. von, 84
Wassermann test, 84
Water, 32, 37, 79, 128–29, 135, 141: in body, 26, 39, 123, 126
Weight, 57: change, 42, 54, 107, 139; control, 31, 37, 122; gain, 13, 37, 49, 123, 124 (fig. 15),

127–29, 139–40, 157, 174, 179, 181, 220; loss, 12–13, 26–27, 37, 39, 87, 123, 157, 213–14
Wheat: germ, 127; whole, 33, 35
Withdrawal: bleeding from the Pill, 49; coitus interruptus, 41, 54; symptoms, from drugs, in infants, 146
Womanly Art of Breastfeeding, 189
Women: black, 183; divorced, 111; heterosexual, 86; Jewish, 99; older (over 30), xi, xvii, 28, 41, 47–48, 51, 90, 107–9, 113, 117–21, 156, 169, 191–92, 200, 228; overweight, 213–14; Rh-negative, 193, 198, 207–8, 214–15; postmenopausal, 243; single, xii, 23, 112; widowed, 111; younger (under 18), 200
Work, xii, 107–8, 110–16, 130–31, 156, 181

X chromosomes, 149 (fig. 16), 150 (fig. 17), 152, 233
X-rays, xii, 24, 94–95, 98, 115–16, 141, 153, 158, 199, 203, 238

Y chromosomes, 149–50 (fig. 17), 152, 233
Yeast infection (moniliasis), 49, 71–73, 216

Zinc, 36, 124–25
Zondek, Bernhardt, 166
Zygote, 250